Healthy Work in an Ageing Europe

Christian Boukal, geb. 1958, Publizistik- und Kommunikationswissenschaftler, Mitarbeiter des Referats Gesundheitsförderung und Vorsorgemedizin der Oberösterreichischen Gebietskrankenkasse in Linz

Oskar Meggeneder, geb. 1945, Soziologe, Sozialökonom und Politikwissenschaftler, Ressortdirektor der Oberösterreichischen Gebietskrankenkasse in Linz, Präsident der Österreichischen Gesellschaft für Public Health

Christian Boukal, Oskar Meggeneder (eds.)

Healthy Work in an Ageing Europe

A European Collection of Measures for Promoting the Health of Ageing Employees at the Workplace

Mabuse-Verlag
Frankfurt am Main

Bibliografische Information Der Deutschen Bibliothek
Die Deutsche Bibliothek verzeichnet diese Publikation in der Deutschen Nationalbibliografie; detaillierte bibliografische Daten sind im Internet unter **http://dnb.ddb.de** abrufbar.

Kasseler Str. 1a
60486 Frankfurt am Main
Tel.: 0 69 / 70 79 96-13
Fax: 0 69 / 70 41 52
www.mabuse-verlag.de

Umschlaggestaltung: Reinhard Koppensteiner, Linz
Layout und Satz: pulpmedia.at, Linz
Englisch: Pat Mallory, Linz
Druck: Prisma Verlagsdruckerei, Frankfurt am Main
ISBN: 3-938304-08-1
Printed in Germany

Contents

Introduction

Christian Boukal, Oskar Meggeneder

The European Network for Workplace Health Promotion (ENWHP) and its initiatives

"Workplace health promotion (WHP) represents the combined efforts of employers, employees and society to improve the health and wellbeing of people at work. This can be achieved by a combination of improving the work organisation and the working environment, promoting active participation and by encouraging personal development." (Luxembourg Declaration 1997)

The 5th Initiative of the European Network for Workplace Health Promotion calls public attention to a special group of workers for the first time.

After some general "Models of Good Practice (MOGP)" of workplace health promotion had been documented (1st Initiative), followed by the implementation of WHP measures in small and medium-sized enterprises (2nd Initiative) and the public administration sector (3rd Initiative), the 4th Initiative turned to the task of analysing and documenting the benefits and effectiveness of WHP measures. The various tools of WHP used in the different partner countries of the Network were described and collected in a "Toolbox". A third aim was to encourage the founding of national WHP forums.

Naturally the partner countries of the Network do not all have the same level of awareness regarding the problems of WHP or its economic benefits. Competition and an entrepreneurial approach to the implementation of WHP occasionally cloud the view of the undeniable benefits it brings. The realisation that both partners in the work process benefit from WHP can easily be obscured when considering the financial investment necessary. Moreover, as could be expected from the title "Workplace Health Promotion", the benefits for the whole of society only become apparent at a later point.

Previous initiatives were geared to awakening interest in WHP in the different stakeholders and describing the benefits for the company, its employees and the whole of society. In this way the ground was prepared for a new view of the connections between work, health and social reality.

WHP follows a holistic approach. For this reason its measures are egalitarian and address persons of both sexes and all ages, companies as well as employees. There is only a difference in approach; between setting-oriented measures and behaviour-oriented measures.

However, ENWHP was unfaithful to this egalitarian principle in the 5th Initiative "Healthy Work in an Ageing Europe" for a very good reason.

By 2030 there will have been a dramatic change in the structure of the population. At present, the 35-45 year olds are in the majority, but in 25 years they will be between 60 and 70 years old and either retired or preparing for retirement.

This biological fact alone will not cause any problems, but together with the declining birth rate of the last 20 years there will be a problem in recruiting qualified workers. More workers will leave working life than will enter it. Many European countries are already facing the problem of how to finance the statutory pension system because of the generous early retirement systems of the past twenty years, which were intended to create jobs for younger workers. If we cannot ensure that more workers enter working life earlier and that the average length of working life is longer, these problems will become even more serious in future, not least because of the constantly increasing life expectancy of our elders.

Although the young people of today are the elders of tomorrow, the 5th Initiative of ENWHP deals solely with workers in the second half of their working lives; these are workers over 45.

The workforce problems which are growing from the demographic change in the European population can be summarised in three statements:

- There will be too few qualified and experienced workers in the future if the current generous pensions system (including early retirement) is continued.
- This means that important knowledge and experience concerning work processes will be lost.
- A dwindling number of workers have to support more retired people through the state transfer system.

Proposed financial changes in the transfer system can only work in the long term and therefore fail to solve the problem in the short term. Higher contributions from workers, lower pensions or models such as one-third financing of pensions through state, company and private means can only function after a long introductory period because confidence in the system must be preserved.

The national state policies therefore are planning to interpret retirement regulations more rigidly and/or to extend working life. Workers who are 45 today must get used to the idea that they will have to work longer than their parents or grandparents did.

This approach to solving the problem needs to be complimented with additional measures if it is to succeed. The general aim is to extend work-ability and health up to a higher age.

This means that both employers and employees will have to take equal responsibility for the health of the workforce. Only then will it be possible to extend working life through improved personal health and a healthier working environment. Workplace health promotion therefore will not merely be an additional measure; it will have to take a central position in company organisation and work processes.

The 5th Initiative will deal with these facts. In many companies, the attitude is that ageing brings deficits, even though it has long been scientifically proved that this is not the case. (Additionally, business complains about the high personnel costs for its older workers if they are paid according to the seniority principle). Various sources stress that ageing does not mean degeneration, but rather a restructuring which has both positive and negative consequences. Although physical abilities decrease with age, mental abilities remain more or less the same. In fact, specialised, mental and social abilities increase with age and can actually be further increased with the right encouragement and challenges.

Using different age groups for different tasks according to their differing capacities and abilities can prevent older workers from being pushed out of the work process and, often enough, into poverty. Workplace health promotion will help to keep older workers at work longer and so help to compensate for the expected lack of qualified workers in the future.

Representatives of workers and employers, the chambers of labour and employers, and, not least, the ENWHP, have therefore long been trying to bring about a change of attitude in companies concerning their human resource policies. The first achievements are becoming visible in some places, although these achievements are mainly restricted to financially strong and labour intensive companies.

Procedure

This report assembles the national chapters on WHP for older workers which is used by the network partners of the ENWHP.

A report was prepared by the project leader to serve as an example. Available material - from internet, from policy papers of the various statutory and private organisations and independent research - was analysed for existing and proposed measures. The information found in this way was collected and converted into a report, which was then given to the ENWHP partners as an example.

This report included:

- The legal basis
- Political aims
- Proposals from:
    - Public services
    - Social insurance institutes
    - Representatives of interest groups
    - Human resource consultants
    - Research organisations
- National projects
- National health promotion policies
- Proposals from different players, for example:
    - Companies
    - Private services (business consultants etc.)
    - Educational institutions
    - Scientific institutions
    - Workplace health promotion organisations (e.g. natio nal and regional forums, national liaison offices, company networks)
- MOGP in each country.

The partners produced their reports according to this example and sent them to the project leader. The national reports were collected in Austria and a table was added to give an overview of the measures. This table is intended to give the reader a quick overview of the different - or similar - measures in the various partner countries.

In order to keep the report a convenient size, the legal basis in the partner countries and the sources have only been published on the CD-ROM which is included. The complete status report of the project "Health Work in an Ageing Europe" is also on the CD-ROM.

As far as the information given allows, the electronic version of the report also provides an active link to the sources cited.

Work, and a satisfying occupation which takes the special abilities of each age group into account, is one of the requirements for healthy ageing. This report shows what possibilities legislators, employers and employees have within their reach.

This report is also available on Internet: www.enwhp.org

Austria

Christian Boukal, Oskar Meggeneder

<table>
<tr><th>Field of promotion</th><th>Physical strain</th><th>Psyche / cognition</th><th>Mental / social competence</th><th>Professional competence</th></tr>
<tr><td>Action</td><td colspan="4"></td></tr>
<tr><td>Relief of physical strain / WHP actions</td><td colspan="2">Setting-based actions</td><td></td><td></td></tr>
<tr><td></td><td colspan="2">Behaviour-based actions *</td><td></td><td></td></tr>
<tr><td></td><td colspan="3">Health circles</td><td></td></tr>
<tr><td></td><td>Reduction of physical strain</td><td colspan="3">Increase in organisational tasks</td></tr>
<tr><td></td><td colspan="3">Promotion and maintainance of physical exercises</td><td></td></tr>
<tr><td></td><td>Micro-breaks</td><td></td><td></td><td></td></tr>
<tr><td></td><td colspan="4">Ageing-friendly work</td></tr>
<tr><td></td><td colspan="4">Extra branches for seniors</td></tr>
<tr><td>Age-related working hours</td><td colspan="2">Reduction of shift work</td><td></td><td></td></tr>
<tr><td></td><td colspan="2">Flexible working hours</td><td></td><td></td></tr>
<tr><td></td><td>Part-time work / flexible pension model</td><td></td><td></td><td></td></tr>
<tr><td></td><td colspan="2">Reduction of night shifts</td><td></td><td></td></tr>
<tr><td></td><td colspan="2">Change in night shift intervals</td><td></td><td></td></tr>
<tr><td>Qualification</td><td></td><td colspan="3">Transfer of knowledge and experience in-company</td></tr>
<tr><td></td><td colspan="4">Age related training for further qualifications</td></tr>
</table>

Fieldloflpromotion	Physicallstrain	Psychel/lcognition	Mentall/lsocial competence	Professional competence
	Better career chances through easier access to qualifications			
Communication		Motivation through participation		
		Increase in mutual appreciation between age groups		
		Improved work operations through better communication and cooperation		
	Change in awareness at management level			
	Coaching for management and personnel			

** Exercise, nutrition, consumption of alcohol and nicotine, relaxation*

Fig.11: Summary of actions - Austria

1. Political basis

The Austrian government is taking measures to promote job security and health for older workers through the Ministries of Business and Labour, and Social Security, Generations and Consumer protection.

1.1. The Federal Ministry of Business and Labour (BMWA)

The Federal Ministry of Business and Labour (BMWA) announced the following measures:

- Wage costs for men over 58 and women over 56 will be reduced by 6 % by discontinuing the contributions to unemployment and accident insurance and also the contributions to the family allowances fund and the insolvency payment fund. The reduction amounts to 12 % for workers over 60.
- A bonus/malus system has been set up for the employment or dismissal of workers over 50. On employment of someone of that age, the employer does not pay any unemployment insurance contribution, on dismissal, a sum of 0.2 % of the last full contribution has to be paid, which can rise to 2.6 times that amount, according to when the dismissal takes place.
- Labour market measures will increasingly be used to train older workers when their job is at risk, and they will have a legal right to such measures after three months unemployment.

1.2. The Federal Ministry for Social Security, Generations and Consumer Protection (BMSG)

In 2004, the Federal Ministry for Social Security, Generations and Consumer Protection (BMSG), together with the federal Chamber of Economy, initiated a competition for enterprises for the state award "Nestor", which was offered under the title of "Maturity Test 2004" (Reifeprüfung). Enterprises successfully implementing measures for "mature" workers were given recognition for their efforts, according to the size of the company. A requirement was that the measures should be set in different fields - on the corporate culture/management level, in personnel policy, motivation, age-friendly working hours and challenges, or workplace health promotion. As well as this, the initiators offered an audit which would provide interested companies with an opportunity to evaluate their measures supporting older workers and to develop them further.

2. National programmes / projects

2.1. The Advice Centre Humane World of Work

The "Advice Centre Humane World of Work" was set up in Austria by the Austrian Social Insurance for Occupational Risks (AUVA) under the title "AEIOU - Retaining Work Ability for Individuals, Organisations and Enterprises" within the scope of the EU initiative EQUAL. Inequality of access to the labour market, because of age, for example, should be evened out by this initiative.

One activity is a study with the title "Preserving and promoting the ability to work", the results of which should enable better use of the different strategies to help older workers retain the ability to work. The study emphasises primary preventative measures.

3. Players

There are numerous players in the field of workplace health promotion in Austria. Several of them are working on proposals for health promotion measures especially for older workers.

These include:

- organisations representing various interest groups,
- private/commercial services, and
- a research institute.

3.1. NGOs / interest group representatives

3.1.1. The Upper Austrian Chamber of Labour (AK OÖ)

The Upper Austrian Chamber of Labour (AK OÖ) is one of the participants in the social partner project "Alter macht Zukunft" (Age makes the Future). This initiative offers the services of two confidential advisors who monitor workplace health promotion projects directly in the enterprise. This ensures that the interests of both employer and employees are considered.

The aim is to discover the potential of ageing employees, to develop it and to use it productively. Additionally, attractive working conditions should be created for them up to retirement, and the health, motivation and training of older workers should be given active support in order to reap the benefits of a workforce consisting of mixed age groups.

Central to the project is an analysis of the enterprise which enables measures to be tailored to the situation. After this "enterprise analysis" the contractors choose the fields of application together with the advisors. Selected project groups then develop solutions with the help of the external advisors, follow them through to the implementation stage and then evaluate them. The structure of the project ensures that the employees play an active role.

According to the social partners, the success of this kind of project for the company and its employees is that:

- knowledge and potential success stays in the company,
- the mutual appreciation of the age groups increases,
- the enterprise improves its image as an employer,
- the employees remain active and motivated up to their retirement because of the attractive working conditions, and
- the available potential is utilised for the benefit of all.The training institute of the Chamber of Labour - Berufsförderungsinstitut (BFI) - offers personal advice and training in matters connected with work, especially for persons over 50.

The topics comprise:

development of further vocational training,
health promotion, and
personal development.

3.1.2. The Chamber of Labour Vienna (AK Wien)

The AK Wien contributes to the website Work and Age (Arbeit und Alter www.arbeitundalter.at) together with the Federation of Austrian Industry (Österreichischen Industriellenvereinigung, see 3.1.5.) and uses it as a databank for successful measures and practical examples.

3.1.3. The Austrian Federal Economic Chamber (WKO)

The Austrian Federal Economic Chamber (Wirtschaftskammer Österreich - WKO) also participates in the project "Age makes the Future" described above, as well as being involved in the "Nestor" award together with the Federal Ministry for Labour and Economy.

Additionally, the WKO's political objectives for its work for older employees are formulated as follows:

- comprehensive, early training and further qualifications for older workers,
- reduction of non-wage labour costs for the employment of older workers,
- evening out of income over the lifetime of employees as the high income of older employees is not sufficiently compensated for by more experience,
- more flexible working hours according to the work ability and life plan of older employees together with a corresponding reduction in payment, and
- information on the special value of workplace health promotion with the project "Age makes the Future" (Alter macht Zukunft).

3.1.4. The Federation of Austrian Trade Unions (ÖGB)

The Federation of Austrian Trade Unions (Österreichische Gewerkschaftsbund - ÖGB) has concrete requirements for an age-friendly organisation of work in an enterprise.

The suggestions are:

- to introduce micro-breaks for older employees,
- to reduce physical demands through re-organisation of work, which can be compensated for by other tasks, such as supervising colleagues,

- to retain the knowledge and experience of older colleagues in the company - in this way the mutual appreciation of the different age groups is increased - , and
- to ensure suitable conditions and a suitable environment for learning for the different age groups.

The Federation offers a "checklist for an ageing-friendly company" on its website. This makes it possible to find out on-line how ageing-friendly the organisation of work is in a company.

3.1.5. The Federation of Austrian Industry (IV)

The Federation of Austrian Industry (IV) has been lobbying for the discontinuation of unemployment insurance contributions for women over 58 and men over 60 (see 1.1.)

Additionally they maintain the informative website Work and Age (Arbeit und Alter www.arbeitundalter.at, see 3.1.2.) together with the Chamber of Labour Vienna. This is a databank of successful examples and international experience and is intended as a virtual consultancy.

Visitors are offered a do-it-yourself check with 26 questions and can find out to what extent ageing-friendly measures are necessary. The evaluation indicates that measures are necessary if the company has insufficient knowledge about the health, motivation and training needs of the employees.

The answers are given individually.

3.2. Private / commercial service enterprises

3.2.1. Institute for Workplace Health Promotion (IBG)

This institute is a commercial consultancy concerned with the dual character of work - its positive and negative effects on health. It offers to set up programmes for human ecology management in enterprises. In "Health Quality Management" (HQM) the correlation between workers interest in work and their ability to accomplish it is shown using validated questions. The resulting figures are shown as "Human Work Index (HWI)" and serve as a management tool in the continuous improvement process of HQM in the independent human ecology management of the enterprise. If there is a high correlation of the factors investigated, there is a salutogenic work situation and the organisation can expect sustainable productivity for the next five years.

Used periodically, the HWI evaluates the results and effects obtained according to a basic survey carried out at the beginning of the programme.

Further elements of HQM are health circles and the health moderation network.

"Productive Ageing" (registered trademark) is a special programme to optimise the job requirements for several generations. The optimal efficiency, meaning of work and work accomplishment should be attained. The aim is to preserve good health up to legal retirement age and beyond.

This is done by utilising the qualities and qualifications of older employees. It is of central importance to take the natural facts of ageing into consideration - physical ability decreases, mental ability stays the same, and both experience and social competence increase. The "Productive Ageing" programme is necessary for many enterprises, according to the IGB, because the age pyramid is reversing or has already reversed, there are fewer people on the labour market and valuable experience and knowledge is being lost to the company through invalidity and early retirement.

"Productive Ageing" programmes promote the potential of ageing employees, sustainably increase the productivity by division of labour between the generations, and facilitate the introduction of new technology which decreases the physical strain of work but requires the mental and social competence that is gained with increasing age.

"Productive Ageing" programmes want to reduce the heavy labour in work and increase the difficulty at the same time. The social inclusion of all the generations in an enterprise should be promoted in the long term. Human ecology personnel management goals are to keep older workers in the company longer, to integrate young workers successfully, to keep knowledge and experience in the organisation, to preserve productive teamwork which includes all the generations and to improve the workplaces ergonomically.

3.2.2. @rbeitsleben (working life)

The private "service partner for workplace health promotion - @rbeitsleben KEG", which is a company from Gmunden, Upper Austria and has branches in Hamburg and Zurich, is participating in the construction of the "Advice Centre Humane World of Work" (Beratungstelle Humane Arbeitswelt) within scope of the EQUAL project AEIOU.

@rbeitsleben's project "Ageing-friendly careers" does not primarily aimto change jobs directly, but wants to effect a change in company organisation and personnel development concepts, which will then allow age(ing) friendly careers to be followed.

The first step is to analyse existing jobs in order to show all the tasks, content, strains, social demands, qualifications required etc.

According to the results, the jobs are categorised as:

- Entry level jobs with short term familiarisation
- Transfer, development or promotion jobs to give a change or for further professional development
- Jobs suited to the age of the workers
- Exit level jobs requiring experienced workers. These jobs have conditions suitable for older workers.

Finding out the strain factor in these categories makes it possible to change job according to health needs and development requirements throughout working life.

A second step entails the evaluation of the jobs by the employees and the design of ageing friendly working careers. At the same time the qualifications and training necessary for these different careers can be determined. After the end of the consultation period, when the aim of "the right work for every age" has been reached, the management should have tools specific to the company in order to carry on working on the continuation of the programme.

3.3. Research organisations

3.3.1. Working Life Research Centre (Forschungs- und Beratungsstelle Arbeitswelt - FORBA)

The Working Life Research Centre (FORBA) works at the point where society, the company and politics meet. Scientific findings on companies, work, technology and gender contribute to improvements in working conditions, especially for older workers.

One of the findings of a study conducted by FORBA has led to the demand for a re-evaluation of the experience of older workers. FORBA also finds "Productive Ageing" projects important.

4. Projects

4.1. Industry

4.1.1. voestalpine AG Linz

This internationally active steel production and manufacturing concern employs a workforce of over 22,000, whereby 14,000 are in Austria. The project "LIFE" aims to reorganise the whole world of work in the concern. The employees should not have to change to suit the work situation; the work situation should change to suit them.

"Formula 33 - further training for all employees" offers the opportunity to spend 2 % of the yearly working time (33 hours) doing training courses.

"Career chances for Elders, too" aims to help remove the barriers which exclude older employees from internal career planning.

"Health and Ergonomics" concerns prophylactic care and the ergonomic design of workplaces.

Work is also being done to reduce night shift work and change the shift pattern for older workers. It has been possible to reduce the sick leave quota considerably through these measures in spite of a rising proportion of older employees.

4.1.2. Agrolinz Melamin

The chemical concern Agrolinz Melamin is a daughter company of the Austrian oil company OMV (Österreichischen Mineralölverwaltung) which has about 1,000 employees. The reorganisation of the company, with redundancies and a stop on recruitment led to an increase in the average age of the workforce. A new model for shift work with 5 shift groups has reduced the weekly working hours from 38 to 34.4. The number of night shifts has been reduced from 8 to 6 and the free shift is now 3-4 days. Every five weeks, one shift is used solely for strategic information and health training. This new organisation required the creation of 50-80 new jobs, which was made possible because the workforce agreed to a pay reduction. The new shift rota was introduced on October 1, 2001.

4.1.3. Polyfelt Linz

Polyfelt is also a daughter company of OMV and produces felts for the underlay of roads. Like Agrolinz Melamin, the working hours per week and the shift interval have been reduced. The workforce agreed to a moderate reduction in pay. The measures increased job satisfaction and the subjective quality of life of those concerned. It also reduced their blood pressure and stress level.

4.1.4. SCA (Schwedische Zellulose AG) Laakirchen

The paper factory Laakirchen has a workforce of 500 of whom two-thirds work shifts with a high level of automation. Together with the works council, the removal of the "catch-up" shift for workers over 50 was achieved. This "catch-up" shift is outside the normal shift rota, and serves only to make the weekly working hours up to 39. The removal of this shift with full remuneration means that the weekly working hours are reduced to 34. Benefits for the company are better work management, higher productivity and a longer working life for the employees, who, of course, are delighted by the changes.

4.1.5. Schmid Schrauben Fabrik Hainfeld (Schmid Screw Factory)

This is a traditional family enterprise with 200 employees, which was taken over by voestalpine after insolvency proceedings. Competition from foreign companies caused the enterprise to concentrate on special orders and innovative solutions. This requires the experience and co-operation of older workers. A high average age and the expected retirement of older workers necessitated the setting up of a knowledge, patent and instrument data bank. A new appreciation of the contributions of older workers to the company was a side effect of this measure.

It also led to both partners reviewing part-time work for older employees, and resulted in a 50 % reduction of daily working time, which is positive for productivity as well as health.

The new insights into the productivity of different age groups increased the respect for older colleagues and thus contributed to their health potential.

4.2. Trade

4.2.1. Food retail and wholesale chain ADEG

The ADEG group, in which the German company EDEKA has majority ownership, has 1,000 branches in Austria and a workforce of 7,500 employees. On May 22, 2002, a supermarket was opened in Bergheim near Salzburg which aims to cater for the needs of older members of the population. It does this by ensuring that price labels can be read easily and goods can easily be reached. Only persons over the age of 50 are employed, recruited exclusively from the long-term unemployed. The idea for "50 +" was given by a customer survey. A further "50+" store has been opened in Vienna, and another is planned for Styria. Special measures for older employees consist of training them in the right way to lift and carry.

4.3. Social Services

4.3.1. Wiener Krankenanstaltverbund (Vienna Hospital Association)

The Vienna Hospital Association is one of the largest health organisations in Europe, with a workforce of over 30,000. Of all the 13,000 nursing employees, only about 1 % work to the regular retirement age, because of the above-average demands made on them. In 1999 the pilot project "Master of Care - an age- and health-friendly career in nursing" was set up to try and prevent staff leaving the profession early because of lack of perspectives and challenges.

The idea is to create a new career stage between nursing and ward management, which is visible both in the job description and in the pay. In future, experienced nurses will take more responsibility for personnel development and internal training on the ward. The model is now in its fourth year and is being tried out and evaluated on three wards of the Vienna Hospitals Association.

4.3.2. Kaiserin Elisabeth Spital des Wiener Krankenanstaltenverbundes (Empress Elisabeth Hospital)

The aim of the project, which ran from 1996 to 2001, was to reduce the daily working time from 12.5 to 8-10 hours a day. The hospital has 280 beds and 700 employees, of whom 300 are nurses. Only 15 % of these are older than 35. The reduced working time for weekdays was introduced on all wards (except the intensive care ward) on October 1, 1996.

An evaluation in 1997 showed a subjective feeling of better health. Overtime was reduced by 44 % in comparison to the previous year, and by a further 17 % in the following year. Sick leave dropped by 30.4 % for the same period of time. The massive dissatisfaction of some of the workforce, who wanted to keep the old 12 hour model, led to the ending of the project in 2001. About 20 % now work shorter shifts on a voluntary basis. The unhealthy long shifts are no longer an unbreakable rule.

4.4. Services

4.4.1. Bankhaus Girocredit

The bank employs a workforce of 2,000 in offices, branches and external work. 1997 "Girocredit Bank AG" was sold and merged with "Erste österreichische Spar-Casse" to become "Erste Bank der österreichischen Sparkassen AG".

At the beginning of the project, half of the workforce was over 40 and enjoyed protection from dismissal. In employees over 50, there was a general lack of motivation and the wish for early retirement. A study of the costs for training and development showed that 95 % of this money was spent on employees under 40, who made up only 55 % of the workforce. The IBG (Institute for Workplace Health Promotion) developed a programme for employees over 40 which concentrated on corporate culture (changing the awareness of the management, meaningful work, and age based alterations to the workplace). It also included coaching for management and employees (for members of management who have age-related problems, for employees in individual crisis situations), and ergonomic measures (easy retirement models, health circles, health promotion with the occupational physician, fitness and nutrition advice).

Great appreciation and enthusiasm for the enterprise were among the results of the evaluation.

Belgium

Veerle Hemans, Karla van den Broek

<table>
<tr><th>Field of promotion</th><th>Physical strain</th><th>Psyche / cognition</th><th>Mental / social competence</th><th>Professional competence</th></tr>
<tr><td>Action</td><td colspan="4"></td></tr>
<tr><td>Relief of physical strain / WHP actions</td><td colspan="2">Setting-based actions</td><td></td><td></td></tr>
<tr><td></td><td colspan="2">Behaviour-based actions *</td><td></td><td></td></tr>
<tr><td></td><td colspan="3">Dynamic risk management (setting, pyschosocial factors, mobbing)</td><td></td></tr>
<tr><td></td><td colspan="4">Task variation / job rotation / mobility between teams</td></tr>
<tr><td></td><td colspan="4">Mentorship for colleagues</td></tr>
<tr><td>Age-related working hours</td><td colspan="2">Time credit</td><td></td><td></td></tr>
<tr><td></td><td colspan="3">Extra holidays for 45+ nurses</td><td></td></tr>
<tr><td></td><td colspan="4">Flexible working hours from certain age on / part-time work / telecommuting</td></tr>
<tr><td></td><td colspan="4">Activaplan</td></tr>
<tr><td></td><td colspan="3">Reduced working hours for 50+ till retirement</td><td></td></tr>
<tr><td>Qualification</td><td colspan="4">Exchange of in-house competences (mentorship, mobility between teams)</td></tr>
<tr><td></td><td></td><td></td><td colspan="2">Survey on demands for training on the job (valorisation)</td></tr>
<tr><td></td><td colspan="4">"Kennispool 50+"</td></tr>
<tr><td></td><td colspan="4">"Experience Fund"</td></tr>
<tr><td></td><td colspan="4">Job-coaching</td></tr>
</table>

<table>
<tr><th>Field of promotion</th><th>Physical strain</th><th>Psyche / cognition</th><th>Mental / social competence</th><th>Professional competence</th></tr>
<tr><td></td><td colspan="4">Kantoor 50+</td></tr>
<tr><td></td><td colspan="4">Career development</td></tr>
<tr><td></td><td colspan="4">Cession of competences to younger colleagues without losses in wage</td></tr>
<tr><td>Communication</td><td colspan="4">Exchange of in-house competences (mentorship, mobility between teams)</td></tr>
<tr><td></td><td></td><td></td><td colspan="2">Improvement of in-house communication</td></tr>
<tr><td></td><td></td><td colspan="3">Improvement of management's competences / corporate culture</td></tr>
<tr><td></td><td></td><td colspan="3">Avoidance of discriminating age-stereotypes / Age-awareness culture</td></tr>
</table>

** Exercise, nutrition, consumption of alcohol and nicotine, relaxation*

Fig. 2: Summary of actions - Belgium

1. Political basis

1.1. The Federal Ministry of Employment and Labour

The Federal Ministry of Employment and Labour guarantees, in a social market economy, the balance of interests between employers and workers in industrial relations. It sees to the protection, the promotion of welfare and to equal opportunities for men and women at work. It contributes actively to the development of the social legislation, both national and international. The Wellbeing Act at Work was introduced in 1996 (August 8, 1996). This act is the Belgian basic act regarding safety and health at the workplace and introduces also other wellbeing domains such as ergonomics, psychosocial issues and industrial hygiene. Most regulations of this act are formulated in the codex of wellbeing at work and are the translation of European regulations or guidelines. Until now, no specific arrangements for elderly workers are mentioned.

Since 2001, a specific fund "Experience Fund" (Ervaringsfonds) has been developed to improve the quality of working conditions of employees older than 55 years. Specific regulations were published in the Royal Decree of January 30, 2003. Initiative comes from the Federal Secretary of Work Organisation and Well-being at Work of the Ministry of Employment and Work. With this fund, companies and sectors are stimulated to develop specific projects for +55ers regarding reorientation, adaptation in the work organisation, education and/or developing an age-awareness culture.

1.2. The Council of Ministers

On November 16, 2004, the Council of Ministers agreed on the preliminary draft of the Programme Law (Programmawet). In this law, specifications regarding the experience fund are mentioned, for example:

- Adaptation from 55 to 45 years, since it is clear that actions to promote better quality of work for elderly workers have to start earlier in the working life.
- Also employees of the public sector have the right to be involved.

- Not only quality of work is important, but also
  - the guarantee of employment (in the own or in another company),
  - psychosocial risks and
  - working time arrangements and payment.
- Sensitisation of the sector and companies is necessary.

To resolve the problems of an older population and consequently increasing social costs, currently a policy is prepared by the federal government in cooperation with the social partners and important organisations (Studiecommissie voor de vergrijzing - Study Committee on Ageing, Hoge raad voor werkgelegenheid - High Council of Employment and Hoge raad voor financiën - High Council of Finance). Specific for the working environment, a longer working life is mentioned in the policy, which draws the attention to quality of life. This policy will result in an action plan for the years 2005-2007.

2. National programmes / projects

2.1. RE-IN +45

This national programme is funded by the EU EQUAL project. It is focused on development and implementation of actions for better integration and reintegration of non-natives and employees over 45 years of age in the labour-market. So far the placement of re-entrants is most possible with large companies, given the feasible prices in the market for small and medium-sized companies (SMEs). Therefore it is necessary to develop a new strategy to place re-entrants in SMEs.

This goal should be obtained via different subgoals:

First the target group of SME has to be identified. Second is identification and selection of adequate occupations for non-natives and older re-entrants, especially those who want to resume work after a phase of inactivity. After these two steps the SMEs need to be convinced to hire from this pool.

Even the target group of the non-native and older unemployed has to be pinpointed. The suggestion is to focus entirely on re-entrants to the labour market - regardless if a non-native or an elder person. Subsequently special information about this group is required: how they could be approached and what their training needs are. The next step would be an individual trajectory corresponding to their respective needs.

In the partnership, representatives of the social partners are present, such as experts from employment organisations and the government. The programme run until the end of 2004.

2.2. Kennispool 50+

VOKA (Kamer van handel van West Vlaanderen, Chamber of Commerce of West Flanders) and the Hogeschool West-Vlaanderen (School of Higher Education West Flanders) developed in 2002 a methodology for knowledge guarantee/transfer. This methodology aims to set up, maintain and transfer the in-house competence. Older employees act as coaches and educators for other teams employed in the same field of work. With support of the Chamber of Commerce and the school specific courses and e-learning tools are developed (Baisier, 2004).

2.3. Silver Instruments and Processes

A team of the Limburgs Universiteit Centrum (LUC) recently introduced a European Social Fund project regarding work motivation and increased availability of older workers. The aim is to organise and develop an age-conscious human resources management in organisations. As a first step the collection of recent projects and initiatives on their website is accomplished.

3. Players

3.1. NGOs / interest group representatives

3.1.1. Federation of Enterprises in Belgium (VBO - Verbond van Belgische Ondernemingen, FEB - Fédération des Entreprises de Belgique)

VBO pinpoints the fact that between 2005 and 2010 the number of potential workers' inflow is less than the potential leavers. Among its suggestions to improve employability are:

- better handling of work reserves (including job seekers, elderly job seekers, fulltime pre-pension workers and fulltime career interruptions). Because unemployed workers tend to be lower educated and are of lesser skills it is very important to pay special attention to issues such as education and training.
- Increasing employability of immigrants.
- Gradually raising the retirement age, implicating a change of institutional rules for early retirement. Working should be promoted versus non-working.
- Better distribution of employment amongst generations and higher retirement pension for a longer working career on the job.

Furthermore the VBO stresses the importance of an age consciousness human resources management. Work protection of elderly workers should be modernised, payment and productivity should be balanced, training improved and the health and well-being policy of the company adjusted to the more specific needs of an ageing workforce. Thus VBO promotes a more active role of the occupational physician regarding medical accompaniment and prevention for elderly workers.

3.1.2. Union of Self-employed (UNIZO - Unie van zelfstandige ondernemers)

The Hoge Raad voor de Werkgelegenheid (High Council of Employment) reveals that the activity rate in Belgium is too low compared with other EU countries, especially regarding +50ers. UNIZO suggests to motivate longer professional careers and to lower the high number of early retirements. This can be done by:

- motivating longer working careers by a bonus in pension payments and thus a reduction in taxes,
- gradually raising the effective retirement age (in SMEs this age generally is already higher than in larger companies), and
- working overtime should be more advantageous for employees, e.g. a tax reduction for working overtime.

The organisation started a service point "KMO en Diversiteit" (SMEs and diversity). It gives free advice and support for the employment of "risk groups": elderly workers, migrant workers and disabled workers. The organisation also gives advice regarding benefits and diversity policy and promotes the development of specific tools and training instruments (e.g. video).

3.1.3. Employees organisations (ACV - CSC - Belgian Christian Trade Union; ABVV - FGTB - Belgian socialist Trade Union; ACLVB - CGSLB - Belgian Liberal Trade Union)

In contrast to the aforementioned opinions both employees organisations - regardless of their political focus - do not share employers' association's point of view regarding the raise of retirement age. But

- current retirement age should be kept (female at 63; male at 65).
- To reject certain discriminations, there should be a right on pre-retirement after a certain career and generalisation of fiscal arrangements (de-cumulation).
- Youngsters, women and non-natives should find better and more opportunities to work.
- Improvement of working conditions especially for older workforces in order to avoid demands for pre-retirement. This could be achieved by changing from shift work to a day job without loss in wages, by improving working conditions, by cutting of working time and by a better education or professional training.

- Extra stimuli for workers who want to work longer than average retirement age (e.g. reemployment with maintenance of the pre-retirement supplement, pension bonus etc.).
- Alternative work-friendly financial agreements (e.g. a general social tax).

3.1.4. Seniorflex

This recently developed organisation wants to unite all active seniors (from 45+) or seniors that want to become active. Their objectives are:

- the right to stay active in a flexible way by combining activity with preservation of social benefits,
- to promote the economical and social value of work for active seniors,
- to sensitise the public opinion and stakeholders, and
- to make a new juridical chapter possible where collaboration is possible.

3.2. Private / commercial service enterprises

3.2.1. SD Worx

Every year SD Worx performs a study regarding job satisfaction and related items. A representative study in 2003 revealed that the Belgian employees desire a retirement age of 55, irrespective of the recent discussion of raising the pension age.

Nevertheless employees remain realistic and make suggestions to increase job and career flexibility in order to solve age problems, e.g. flexible working hours, work at home.

The study gives an important proposal to human resources departments: improve communication with the older workers in search of best solutions.

3.2.2. Employment agencies:

3.2.2.1. Governmental:

- Vlaamse Dienst voor Arbeidsbemiddeling en Beroepsopleiding (VDAB),
- le service public wallon de l'emploi et de la formation professionnelle (FOREM) and

- Office Régional Bruxellois de l'Emploi (ORBEM) are governmental (Flemish, Walloon and Brussels) agencies for unemployment engaged with job-coaching, consultancy and training

3.2.2.2. Private interim agencies (e.g. t-interim)

Several initiatives exist in the employment agencies to support older workers. Some examples:

- *Jobcoaching:* support for specific populations (+45ers, non-native workers or disabled persons) during the job application procedure and integration in the working field up to six months after employment. The applicant receives a special job coaching contract to promote a smooth integration in a company.
- *Activaplan:* support is given to employers to introduce the diversity policy in the company by a decrease of employer's contribution for the recruitment of elderly work-seekers (the so-called Activaplan).
- *Kantoor 45+ (Office 45+):* a specific interim agency with the objective to help people older than 45 to find a job (t-interim; private interim agency). Therefore a thorough conversation about motivation, ambition and work expectance is conducted. The consultant searches job vacancies regarding the work possibilities and contacts companies to promote the older worker and to explain the benefits of the applicant.
- *Mentorship:* a mentor is a more experienced individual (often older workers) willing to share his/her knowledge with someone less experienced in a relationship of mutual trust. Specific mentor training programs exist to teach the future mentor how to transfer knowledge and how to improve professional, teaching and relational competences (VDAB).

CEFORA: Centre de Formation de la CPNAE (Commission Paritaire Nationale Auxiliare pour Employés)

The CHECK-UP 45+ methodology was created. The methodology makes a valorisation of the older workers' qualities. A competencies analysis is made regarding further development of these workers in their company. Recommendations regarding training and/or new job possibilities are given.

3.3. Research organisations

3.3.1. Flemish Social-Economic Council (De Sociaal-Economische Raad van Vlaanderen - SERV) Flemish Technological Foundation (Stichting Technologie Vlaanderen STV)

STV - Innovation & Work is a research institute of the Flemish Social Partners (SERV) and financed each year by the Flemish government.

The institute recently published the results of the study "Employability of the older worker: experiences of HR management" ("De tewerkstelling van oudere werknemers: ervaringen van HR-managers", 2004). Reflections on age-conscious human resources policy are given and the translation of the policy in practice is discussed. The policy includes meetings regarding function expectations, competent management, career support, training and coaching and is considered as a tool to keep and increase the employability of employees in a company in accordance with the needs and expectations of different age groups.

Another publication of this research institute addresses the indicators of work quality in the Flemish working environment ("Vlaamse Werkbaarheidsmonitor", Bourdeaud'hui et al. 2004). Work stress, task variation, support from direct supervisors and working conditions were mentioned as important variables that differ between younger and older workers.

3.3.2. Prevent

Prevent, institute for occupational safety and health, analysed in cooperation with VUB (Free university of Brussels, Faculty of Psychology and Educational Sciences, 2004), the Belgian results of the study of the European Foundation for Living and Working Conditions regarding working conditions (Paoli, 2003). In this report small differences were reported with age groups regarding physical working conditions, risk awareness, and the relation between work and health problems.

4. Projects

4.1. Industry

4.1.1. Volvo Cars

The car manufacturer employs 5,000 people in Gent. The company supports mobility between teams and departments and expresses the importance of the older worker.

During internal job recruitments, experience is an important issue. Experience and seniority are decisive preconditions for staffing. This strategy keeps older workers in the company and guarantees new challenges for younger employees, since they can take up the former jobs of older staff members.

The company performs a lot of effort in ergonomic working conditions which affect all employees.

Job rotation is promoted so that there is a variety of physical tasks.

Specific adapted workstations with low physical challenge exist (e.g. control jobs). These positions are kept for people who are in need of them (e.g. persons with disabilities, elder workers with restricted physical possibilities etc.).

Often older workers function as mentors for younger workers and train them on the job.

4.1.2. Company X (company wants to stay anonymous)

The company manufactures steal wire and employs 4,372 person at 15 locations in Belgium. In Zwevegem more than 40 % of 2,400 employees are older than 45 years. About 200 workers are older than 50 years and are working with the time credit system. 1,947 are pre-retirement workers.

About 2,000 employees left the company after three reorganisations, mainly via pre-retirement arrangements. As a result much in-house competence vanished and production figures dropped over a period of two years. Therefore extra training had to be provided for younger employees.

These circumstances led to more age consciousness in the human resources management.

Older employees obtained an exemplary function in their positions and further career perspectives were given. Younger employees are therefore disposed for lifelong training on the job and taking an active part in their career management to be sure of keeping their job.

If higher management personnel is confronted with age related problems, the possibility to cut responsibilities and remain in a "weakened" version of their function was created.

For workers most problems are related to shift work. The company tried to work with a fixed night shift schedule, but this was cancelled due to communication problems.

In selection procedures of new candidates, discrimination was abolished since age-oriented criteria are no longer of interest, whereas competencies are emphasised.

4.1.3. Egemin

610 employees in Belgium produce technological and automatic solutions for the distribution of raw materials used in the nutrition, pharmaceutical and distribution sector and in warehousing applications.

To follow and structure the growth of the company, an innovative human resources policy is kept. One of the important topics was the search for experienced +50 workers on the labour market since the management was convinced of the invaluable source of information and know-how that these people can bring into the company. Today for 10 younger workers there is a worker older than 48. They transfer their experience to the highly educated young worker that has insufficient methodic knowledge. This results in a very fruitful cooperation that positively effects both parties.

4.2. Social services

4.2.1. UZ Leuven

The university hospital of Leuven employs a workforce of 8,000, including a nursing staff of 2,600 at the average age of 40.5 years. Almost one third is 45 years or older. A specific collective work agreement exists for nurses regarding working hours reduction: +45ers have on extra holiday each month, +50ers two days and +55ers three days. Although it is generally preferred to retire early, the hospital gains achievements in creating good work situations. A commission was installed for prevention of lower back problems by providing back training, ergonomic helping devices etc.

Furthermore, experienced employees can become mentors that accompany and teach trainees and beginners.

4.3. Services

4.3.1. Company Y (company wants to stay anonymous)

The company is a bank/insurance group for private and medium-sized companies and gives work to 16,000 employees in Belgium.

Pre-retirement arrangements did cut the age-group older than 50 years significantly, whereas there are many 40-50ers.

The company tries to implement more age consciousness in its human resources system in favour of the entire staff, but nevertheless places specific emphasis on problems of elderly workers.

The company promotes changes in corporate culture and strongly rejects to stereotype characteristics regarding older employees.

Based on staff interviews it became clear that older employees got problems with new types of office work (less administrative work, more front desk work which demands new relational and commercial skills). Increasing computer work and the increasing amount of new specific services and products were also mentioned as problem areas.

Therefore the bank at the moment does a survey on how to improve the situation via several selective initiatives: shift of older employees to other functions without loss of acquired function-specific advantages, yearly evaluations, career development and support as well as time credit systems.

Czech Republic

Alena Steflova

<table>
<tr><th>Field of promotion</th><th>Physical strain</th><th>Psyche / cognition</th><th>Mental / social competence</th><th>Professional competence</th></tr>
<tr><td>Action</td><td colspan="4"></td></tr>
<tr><td>Relief of physical strain / WHP actions</td><td colspan="2">Setting-based measures</td><td></td><td></td></tr>
<tr><td></td><td colspan="2">Behaviour-based measures *</td><td></td><td></td></tr>
<tr><td></td><td colspan="2">Screening for occupational risks and deseases</td><td></td><td></td></tr>
<tr><td></td><td colspan="3">Early medical screening</td><td></td></tr>
<tr><td></td><td colspan="4">New corporate culture favouring teamwork</td></tr>
<tr><td></td><td colspan="4">"Mentoring" of younger by older employees</td></tr>
<tr><td></td><td>Back exercises, physiotherapy</td><td></td><td></td><td></td></tr>
<tr><td></td><td colspan="4">Anti-stress programmes for managers</td></tr>
<tr><td></td><td colspan="3">Improving working conditions and work environment</td><td></td></tr>
<tr><td>Age-related working hours</td><td colspan="2">Supportive exit strategies</td><td></td><td></td></tr>
<tr><td>Qualification</td><td colspan="4">Supportive infrastructure for continued training and qualification</td></tr>
<tr><td></td><td colspan="4">Creation of new educational tools, i.e. lifelong learning</td></tr>
<tr><td></td><td colspan="4">Improving the quality of managerial staff and processes</td></tr>
<tr><td>Communication</td><td></td><td colspan="3">Supporting interpersonal relationship</td></tr>
<tr><td></td><td></td><td colspan="3">Counselling and introduction of new staff</td></tr>
</table>

Field of promotion	Physical strain	Psyche / cognition	Mental / social competence	Professional competence
		Developing reference indicators for effectiveness of health promotion measures		
		Counselling and assistance for entrepreneurial health promotion programmes		
		Distribution of know-how relating to WHP - methodological support for employers		
		Regular seminars focused on ageing and older workers		
		Programmes promoting health apart from work (incl. families)		

** Exercise, nutrition, consumption of alcohol and nicotine, relaxation*

Fig. 3: Summary of actions - Czech Republic

1. Political basis

State Authorities:

1.1. Ministry of Health (MoH)

Controls the following authorities:
- State Health Institute (SHI)
- Institute of Health Informatics and Statistics (IHIS)

The MoH's formulation of national health policy is based on agreements, declarations and recommendations by the United Nations Organisation (UNO), World Health Organisation (WHO) and European Council (EC). Their principal document in the Czech Republic is entitled "Health for All in the 21st Century". The implementation of the "Agreement on Human Rights and Dignity Protection" is also of high importance, especially concerning biological and medical terms.

The WHO programme "Health for All in the 21st Century" is implemented in the "Long-term Programme for the improvement of the Health Status of the Population in CR - Health for All in the 21st Century", which is the elaboration of the WHO strategy, adopted by the Czech government in Decision No. 1046 from October 30, 2002.

It focuses on the training of handicapped and chronically ill persons, achieving higher levels of efficiency in medical treatment, higher quality of life for disabled persons and saving federal budget expenses. The management, coordination and control of tasks related to this programme are guaranteed by the Health and Environment Board, which established a special "Committee of Health 21" to prepare proposals, papers and tasks.

The Ministry of Health is collaborating with the Ministry of Labour and Social Affairs on joint efforts in both the sectors "ageing and health care" and "social service coordination". The main strategy of the health care sector aims at improving the health status of fellow citizens, notably the protection and promotion of health, by
- putting the patient at the centre of health service delivery and thus strengthening the patient's own responsibility for his health,

- improving basic health status indicators while cutting the number of the most frequent diseases and the risk factors which may be contributing to their increase,
- improving the quality of life for elders, and
- encouraging intersectoral cooperation in different political realms to promote health and to prevent illnesses.

Demographic development forced the MoH to adopt a specific grant programme as an instrument for promoting a solution to the age problem. This is a concrete contribution by the ministry to accomplishing the "National programme for the preparation for ageing 2003-2007". Referring especially to seniors, the programme "Health for All in the 21st Century" of the MoH aims at the following targets:

- increasing the number of years spent in good health,
- promoting an active and fulfilled social life,
- prolonging life and the quality of life by improving life style and creating a motivating environment.

1.2. Ministry of Labour and Social Affairs (MLSA)

Controls the following authorities:

- Research Institute of Labour and Social Affairs
- Institute of Labour Safety Education
- Research Institute of Labour Safety
- Offices of Labour - regional

Historically, the Czech Republic is an advanced industrial country in which industry contributes 32.9 % of the GDP. Approximately 26 % of the total workforce is employed in industry. The Ministry of Industry and Trade collaborates with the Ministry for Regional Development (MfRD) on the formation and negotiation of the successful National Plan of Development for the Republic. The European Social Fund (ESF) is one of the structural instruments of the EU supporting the European Strategy of Employment (ESE) which has the target of improving the employment rate and work ability of workers within the European Union.

Analysis of human resource development - including qualification requirements - has shown certain setbacks in the field of human resource policy in industry. The priority of federal employment policy is to focus on groups endangered by long-term unemployment, which has proved to be good practice. Elderly employees are the group endangered most by social exclusion and hence great attention has to be paid to them.

A sectoral operational programme of the European Union Human Resources (MLSA) proposed to introduce measures to overcome setbacks which had been identified. In addition, specific measures of a Sectoral Operational Programme of the Ministry of Industry and Trade (MIT) give support to infrastructure for continued vocational training and improvement of qualifications. Better utilisation of human resources is the long-term aim, including risk-groups, e.g. older employees.

As far as support from structural funds is addressed, from reasons mentioned above, areas benefiting are as follows:

- Support in the foundation and development of small and medium-sized enterprises, development of business and business services, development of infrastructure for transport and coverage of area service as well as support for direct international investments.
- Better utilisation of manpower, creation of new working opportunities and development of the industry's human resources for to improve competitive ability. These tasks should be accomplished by measures for monitoring of Sector Operational Programmes (SOP), currently being implemented.
- Overcoming inequalities and thus promoting equality between the sexes, among the unemployed population (caused by both social exclusion and age structure), promotion of all employment trends, enhancement of qualification levels for human potential.

Both the operational programme and the rules for participation in this programme promote equal chances for all the subjects targeted. Very important components of these programmes are care for employees and their working environment as well as continuous health care.

Interventions for achieving equality of opportunity will be regularly monitored and assessed regarding their results, especially those benefiting from structural funds. One criterion is, for example, the number of newly employed women out of total number of newly created jobs in the industrial sector. From the results of these checks, conclusions for further efficient measures could be made to set the principle of equal opportunities in promoting respective policies and measures. Currently only first proposals were submitted to the Minister of Regional Development as SOPs are in the very beginning.

For the future, efficient human resources policies will also be based on support for the creation of educational and training centres within enterprises (special workshops, laboratories, teaching rooms etc.). Facilities which extend beyond regional activities, building up company education systems which especially encourage distance and electronic learning (e-learning), promoting workers' acquaintance with the global information society will receive assistance. Furthermore, the creation of educational tools and programmes, workshops and seminars, and consultancy leading to a better personnel policy as well as a higher quality of managerial staff and processes is targeted.

The measures will focus on necessary training structures - above all in small and medium-sized enterprises. The development of consulting services for enterprises' management of human resources will be supported, especially short-term managerial education, tailor-made to the real demands of enterprises.

1.3. Ministry of Industry and Trade (MIT)

1.4. Ministry for Regional Development (MfRD)

1.5. Ministry of Finance (MoF)

1.6. Trade Unions

- Czech-Moravian Confederation of Trade Unions
- Association of Independent Trade Unions

1.7. Health Insurance Funds (HIF)

- General Health Insurance Company (GHIC).
- Further Branch Health Insurance Companies unified in Health Insurance Companies Union with state range activity: Military HIC, HIC of MoI, Branch HIC.

- With regional activity range: Metallurgical HIC, Škoda HIC, METAL/ALLIANCE HIC, Czech National HIC - CNHIC, Miner Brothers HIC - MBHIC.

2. National programmes / projects

Programme documents of the Czech Republic and relevant basic principles adopted in EU are included especially in:

- regulation of the European Council (EC) No. 1260/99 on general provisions of Structural Funds,
- regulation of the European Parliament and the European Council (EC) No. 1261/99 on European Fund of Regional Development,
- regulation of the European Parliament and the European Council (EC) No. 1784/99 on European Social Fund (ESF) and
- regulation of the European Council (EC) No. 1447/2001, amending Regulation of European Council (EC) No. 1260/1999 on general provisions of Structural Funds.

The European Strategy on Employment defines four pillars: employment, promotion of enterprises, adaptability and equal chances. The European Social Fund concentrates on five political areas in the period from 2000-2006, according to the pillars of the European Strategy of Employment. These areas are:

- active labour market policy,
- equal chances for access to the labour market,
- life-long education,
- improvement of women's access, and
- participation of women in the labour market.

The harmony of the European Strategy of Employment and of the Czech National Action Plan of Employment will be supported, above all, by the ESF by means of the Sectoral Operational Programme (SOP) - Human

Resources Development. Connection of SOP - Industry and Enterprise and SOP - Human Resources Development, based on highly qualified and flexible working power will achieve the necessary synergetic effects.

2.1. "Health for All in the 21st Century" (hereinafter Health 21)

An important Health 21 objective is the reduction of existing differences in the health status within countries as well as among European states. This difference is an element of social inequality and a factor that may negatively influence the stability of national communities and, consequently, the overall region. From this standpoint, the Czech population is not afflicted with an alarming health status; however, problems are not totally absent. In spite of significant progress, the republic has also not yet reached the health parameters of the most developed industrial countries in Western democracy. However, the level of health is substantially dynamic in time and both the potential and actual health status of individuals and the population are constantly moving upwards, as in many prosperous societies.

Health 21 puts great emphasis on the participation of all members of society in improving national health and on the shared responsibility of all official bodies. Recognising health as a specific motive and an occasion for cooperation between government departments and a criterion for political decision-making has not yet become common practice within Czech ministries. This mainly concerns the impact on health of key decisions concerning the generation of power, transportation, legislation, agriculture, education and taxation. It is known that access to public transport significantly influences access to health care, that the content and level of education strongly determine attitudes towards health and a person's social environment is decisive for his state of health. Some countries have already made health impact assessment subject to their strategic decisions. Health 21 formulates two specific targets focused on ageing population and health promotion at workplaces.

Target 5: Healthy Ageing

By the year 2020, people over 65 years should have the opportunity of enjoying their full health potential and playing an active social role.

Specific target 5.1: There should be an increase of at least 20 % in life expectancy and in disability-free life expectancy at the age of 65 years achieved step by step according to partial targets and instruments formulated in Health 21 (settled by Government decree No. 1046/2002).

Target 13: Settings for Health

By the year 2015, people should have greater opportunities to live in healthy social and economic environments at home, at school, at the workplace and in local communities.

Specific target 13.6: Ensuring that at least 10 % of medium and large-sized companies commit themselves to healthy company/enterprise principles.

As far as workplaces are concerned, this target is not limited to reducing risk factors but also encourages employees' and employers' participation in creating a safer and healthier working environment as well as reducing stress at work. Every company should specify targets of the Health 21 programme according to its own terms by jointly identifying goals and measures. In addition to prevention and treatment of injury, programmes should also address broader lifestyle and environmental issues and promote a company culture favouring teamwork and open discussion of problems, including the special issue of older workers.

A good example of inter-sectoral cooperation in the Czech Republic is the National Environment Health Action Plan. However, it needs to be further developed and more intensely applied at regional and local levels. Analogous to the principles of the Health 21 document are the provisions of Article 152 of the European Union's Amsterdam Treaty, which states, "a high level of human health needs to be incorporated in all policies and strategies of the European Communities". Health 21 respects all previously approved documents relevant to the population's health status, such as the State Environmental Policy, the Transportation Policy and the Energy Policy.

3. Players

3.1. Health Insurance Companies (HIC)

- General Health Insurance Company (GHIC).
- Further Branch Health Insurance Companies unified in the Health Insurance Companies Union with a state range of activity: Military HIC, HIC of MoI, Branch HIC.
- Companies with a regional range of activity: Metallurgical HIC, Škoda HIC, METAL/ALLIANCE HIC, Czech National HIC - CNHIC, Miner Brothers HIC - MBHIC.

Health insurance companies contribute to the organisation and implementation of preventive programmes. They mediate preventive health care at company level but also try to motivate both entrepreneurs and individual insurees to participate in health promotion programmes. HICs evaluate these programmes together with those employers and employees involved.

To prevent diseases of older groups of insured persons, instructions leading to increased physical activity, early cardiovascular and oncological screening, stomatological prevention and decrease of pain related to the musculo-skeletal system are of high value and importance.

3.2. NGOs

3.2.1. The Forum of Health Promoting Organisations of the Czech Republic (hereinafter Forum)

The Forum was established in 2002 as an association of legal entities, holding its first general assembly in October 2003. Any legal entity accepting the obligations stipulated in the Forum's statutes and supporting the targets of the association may become a member. Membership to the association underlines the will to support the strategy of the European Union (ENWHP) and of the World Health Organisation (WHO/EURO), to launch projects of health promotion and improvement of life style, and to actively search for and promote sustainable developments of health and quality of life by implementing a comprehensive health, environment and work safety management.

Relating to all these activities the association's members are obliged to further primary disease prevention and promote the development and dissemination of knowledge about workplace health so that private and working life are conducive to good health. Moreover they should aim to modify unhealthy habits and behaviour at workplaces, and support interpersonal relationships as well as corporate culture and prosperity.

The task of the Forum is to integrate interested stakeholders on an unofficial basis and to direct enterprises to greater responsibility for their employees' health.

3.2.2. The Consortium for Health Promotion and the Primary Prevention of Diseases (hereinafter Consortium)

In 2003, the Ministry of Interior approved the Code of the Consortium as an independent agency of the above Forum. Its educational activities are based on scientifically justified principles of health promotion. The Consortium facilitates the inclusion of the research and teaching staff of five universities in the Czech Republic and intends to decentralise the educational programme, taking it out into the administrative regions, so that WHP projects can be more effectively introduced in these regions.

The Forum cooperates with the Consortium to foster educational courses, advisory seminars and training, and provides information on proven methods, programmes and tools. This also includes counselling and assistance in launching health promotion projects as well as regional promotion. Negotiations with strategic national and international partners are also part of the service provided. Assimilating and distributing information about intervention and behaviour modification, and also providing methodological support for employers as well as trade unions are further aims.

The association provides these services either through its own employees or by third party professionals. In 2003, the Forum's information and educational programme on the Internet (www.forumZPO.cz) was set up. The translation and publication of D. Chenoweth´s book "Workplace Health Promotion" was another important activity within the Consortium (its second part "Workplace Health Promotion Projects Evaluation" focused on cost-effectiveness). The organisation of three national conferences entitled "Towards a Good Practice in Health, Safety and Environment in Enterprises - HESME" also provided a platform for stakeholders and all parties involved in this process, such as employers' associations, labour unions, health insurers, federal and public administration bodies as well as non-profit organisations. A further task of this NGO body is the dissemination of the 5th ENWHP initiative focused on the topic of the ageing workforce.

3.2.3. GEMA

GEMA is a non-governmental organisation focused on health of older people which supports the interlinking of health care and promotion, social care, safety, scientific institutions, media, employers etc. with the aim of creating comprehensive geriatric assessment and an approach to the needs of older people. It facilitates the cooperation of federal and public administration bodies as well as non-profit organisations and insurers in this process. One of the activities is the realisation of the project "Healthy Ageing in the Czech Republic".

The elderly population - being very heterogeneous in terms of health status and functional ability - requires differentiated approaches and projects. Only a minority of seniors lose their autonomy, which is always a result of a combination of disability, environmental obstacles and social situations (loneliness being an especially significant factor).

Examples of some specific health promotion activities to achieve certain targets are:

- reducing the cardiovascular diseases - checking symptoms and risk factors of atherogenesis in middle age,
- reducing the prevalence of injuries - health education programmes to increase safety of environments, rehabilitation and physiotherapeutic programmes, healthy lifestyle,
- improving the effectiveness and usefulness of health services for seniors - geriatric modification of existing services and
- supporting programmes of NGOs active in the area of sports that focus on physical activity of the ageing population.

The location of the organisation - Gerontocentrum, Prague 8.

3.3. Private / commercial service enterprises

3.3.1. PREMEDIS s.r.o., Liberec

PREMEDIS is a private service focused on health promotion at work on regional level (Liberec region). Its activities not only address prevention and treatment of occupational risks and diseases but also broader issues of healthy lifestyle and environments. Measures of intervention are focused on individuals as well as on groups of employees, including relevant age groups.

3.3.2. KARDIA, Prague

This private service is oriented towards occupational preventive care focusing on healthy lifestyle issues and intervention based on the assessment of specific needs of employees. It encourages efforts to increase employees' and employers' participation in creating a healthier environment. The organisation possesses agencies in several cities of the Czech Republic.

3.4. Research organisations

3.4.1. National Institute of Public Health:

The Institute's research plan "Analysis of infections, environmental and behavioural health risks and their prevention" is divided to four partial research topics, which are conducted within 35 research projects:

- analysis of behavioural health risks and their prevention,
- prevention, diagnosis and therapy of serious, new or newly occurring communicable diseases,
- environmental health risks assessment, and
- assessment of health risk factors in occupational environments.

Recent findings and suggestions of the National Health Institute's research plan are related to an increasing awareness of behavioural and social factors (determinants) in health - being a new paradigm in the research of this institute as well as in Czech society.

One of the centres of this institute is Centre of Industrial Hygiene and Occupational Health. This centre creates the basic conditions for the study of problems associated with industrial medicine, including basic and applied research. Centre is also active in area of promotion of health in the workplaces.

3.4.2. Occupational Safety Research Institute (VÚBP)

VÚBP is a contributory organisation run by the Ministry of Labour and Social Affairs.

The mission of VÚBP is the research and development of means to reduce the risks involved in work activities and increase efficiency in production, work culture and work satisfaction.

The main topics are:

- monitoring and foreseeing trends in workplace safety and health protection,
- a comprehensive and systemic approach, and
- the quality of services and products (protective tools and measures).

The policies of VÚBP are based on a systemic approach to the prevention of hazards to human health and life and dangers to environment and property, which are inherent in economic (work) activities.

VÚBP particularly focuses on the support of system changes and the institute's policies, methods and applications are considered to cover this aim to a notable extent. This implies a wide support in the performance of work safety tasks by government authorities, especially in defining and testing the government's policy in compliance with Convention No. 155/1981 ILO. At present VÚBP is not focused on seniors. However, the institute is part of a network of occupational health promotion, and senior issues will be dealt with in the near future.

An important factor behind the institute's activities is the fulfilment of requirements set out in an "Association Agreement" with the EU and the preparation for the Czech Republic's accession to the EU. Therefore, VÚBP is expanding and intensifying its activities in standardisation, testing and certification, especially regarding technical standardisation and the testing of products in regulated areas. The Science and Research (S&R) policy concerning workplace safety is based on the Czech Republic's social doctrine which regards the provision of satisfying and safe working conditions as an integral part of the country's social policy. It follows up on the National Policy, the Ministry of Labour and Social Affairs' S&R policy and the Institute's research project "Means and Instruments of Increasing Occupational Safety Levels" implemented in 2000-2003, defining and determining basic research objectives regarding workplace safety.

The goal of the above policy is to research, design and verify measures aimed at ensuring permanent improvements in safety and efficiency of work as well as corporate culture.

4. Projects

4.1. "Healthy Company Project"

In 1995, based on the relevant WHO/EURO initiative, the Czech Ministry of Health (MoH) entrusted the "National Network for Health Promotion in the Workplace" with realising the "Healthy Company Project" that was set out in the MoH's strategic programme approved by the Czech Government in its Resolution 273/1992. Health promotion provides health protection activities in companies with a new concept of health education. However, unlike occupational health and safety, practising health promotion at work is not required by laws or other regulations and therefore remains an "above-standard" action. But the required infrastructure is still weak and what is especially lacking are incentives by federal administration bodies to motivate enterprises.

The first national conference on "Good Practice in Health, Environment and Safety Management in Industrial and Other Enterprises", held in 1999, was a step towards the implementation of health promotion programmes in workplaces. It pointed out necessary tasks for the future, such as legislative proposals concerning taxes that will take more account of health protection and promotion. Moreover it proposed to reinforce incentives for companies linked to health, sickness and accident insurance which should also help achieve these objectives. Other tasks are the development of reference indicators for effectiveness, conducting training and education for professionals in health promotion, setting up a network of counselling services, and identifying needs for the preparation and implementation of regional and local health promotion programmes. These tasks are being very slowly performed in cooperation with the ministries responsible, especially the MoH and MoLSA, and the representatives of both employers and employees.

4.2. Projects implemented in companies

The projects of health promotion at workplaces are implemented in companies which are winners of the Healthy Company Award. These companies are members of the National Forum of Health Promoting Organisations. Other interested companies use their experience, especially in terms of management and the positive influence on employees, as examples of good practice for broader implementation of health promotion programmes in the Czech Republic.

Running projects:

Škoda Auto a.s. Mladá Boleslav

The Volkswagen company of Mlada Boleslav is a leading company in WHP in the Czech Republic, including WHP for seniors. Having good sources from the mother company in Germany it can relatively easily put new aspects of WHP into practice.

At present, other companies are only in the very beginning of the development of WHP procedures focused on seniors.

Energetické a ekologické stavitelství - závod Zeleznicní stavby Brno
Ceská rafinérská a.s. Litvínov
Severomoravská energetika a.s. Ostrava
CEZ, a.s., Jaderné elektrárny Temelín a Dukovany
Nová huc a.s.- Ostrava - Kuncice
Procter+Gamble - Rakona, a.s.
EASTMAN Sokolov a.s.
Všeobecná zdravotní pojištovna
ZP Metal-Aliance
Hutnická pojištovna Ostrava

Project activities of the above mentioned "Healthy Companies" include:

- A safer working environment, including the prevention and control of physical hazards and screening for occupational risks and diseases.
- An improved attitude towards meals in the factory canteen and towards non-smoking policy. Participation in screening programmes (breast cancer screening, colo-rectal carcinoma screening).
- Vaccination (flu, tick encephalitis), vitamin supply etc.
- Activities oriented to the recovery of manpower, such as physiotherapy and the renewal of physical fitness (project "Back Exercise").

- Programmes to promote health outside work (relaxing stay in a spa, physical activities and other sport activities for the entire family etc.).
- Anti-stress programmes (mostly for managers).
- Initiatives to address psychosocial risk factors at workplaces, such as offering counselling, the introduction of new staff, "mentoring" by older staff or supportive exit strategies.

On the basis of the available information some conclusions can be drawn by assessing supplied data to map the current situation in other companies. Up to now, Czech enterprises which are executing health promotion activities are predominantly production plants, chiefly with 100-400 employees. Most of these activities are financed by the companies themselves, sometimes with the co-participation of the state (on the basis of a grant system), or by health insurance companies. The most frequent health promotion actions are attempts to influence nutrition habits via company catering and activities against nicotine abuse. Actions against alcohol and drug abuse are implemented less frequently.

Another group of preventive activities can be labelled as "labour risks and their limitation" and these address the improvement of working conditions and environment. Predominant in this respect are preventive medical checkups for employees working in so-called "hazardous workplaces". This is in full accordance with the prevailing national attitude towards workplace health as well as with the legal concept of employees' welfare. Nevertheless, there is an increasing number of companies which pay attention not only to the limitation of common labour risks but also to well-known factors that may have a negative impact on employees' health.

4.3. Model and pilot projects

4.3.1.

The model project proposal of General Health Insurance Sokolov - for health promotion, screening, intervention and primary prevention.

Realisation of the project is planned in 2003-2006.

Guarantors: General Health Insurance Sokolov - Ivan Gajewski, M.D., Jana Kocianová, M.D.

4.3.2.

The model regional project: "Health care strategy in the companies of Liberec Region". The project supports the interlinking of health promotion, occupational health care and work safety creating a comprehensive and coordinated system of management and education in this area.

Guarantors: Premedis s.r.o. - Tatjana Šoltysová. Regional Hygienic Station of Liberec Region - M.D., Vladimir Valenta, M.D.

4.3.3.

Project "Employment and active lifestyle" - organises regular seminars especially focused on ageing and older workers.

Guarantor: The Czech Association of Occupational Psychologists and Managers (CAPPO).

4.3.4.

Project "Healthy Ageing in the Czech Republic" - a comprehensive approach to the needs of older people.

Coordinator: NGO GEMA, Iva Holmerova, M.D., Gerontocentrum, Prague 8.

Denmark

Kurt Æbelø, Ervin Jensen

<table>
<tr><th>Field of promotion</th><th>Physical strain</th><th>Psyche / cognition</th><th>Mental / social competence</th><th>Professional competence</th></tr>
<tr><td>Action</td><td></td><td></td><td></td><td></td></tr>
<tr><td>Relief of physical strain / WHP actions</td><td colspan="2">WHP measures *</td><td></td><td></td></tr>
<tr><td></td><td colspan="2">Promoting healthy lifestyle</td><td></td><td></td></tr>
<tr><td></td><td colspan="3">Check of individual working fitness</td><td></td></tr>
<tr><td></td><td colspan="4">Flexible tasks for seniors</td></tr>
<tr><td></td><td colspan="2">Transfer to less demanding positions</td><td></td><td></td></tr>
<tr><td></td><td colspan="4">Senior policy and working environment matching physical attrition and abilities of older workers</td></tr>
<tr><td></td><td colspan="3">Developing a good physical and psychological working environment</td><td></td></tr>
<tr><td>Age-related working hours</td><td colspan="3">Flexible working hours for seniors</td><td></td></tr>
<tr><td></td><td colspan="2">Part-time employment</td><td></td><td></td></tr>
<tr><td></td><td colspan="2">Less working hours for seniors</td><td></td><td></td></tr>
<tr><td></td><td colspan="4">Individual senior schemes (positions, working hours)</td></tr>
<tr><td></td><td colspan="4">Special employment contracts for seniors (working time, early retirement, future pensions etc.)</td></tr>
<tr><td>Qualification</td><td></td><td colspan="3">Continued training and upgrading</td></tr>
<tr><td></td><td></td><td colspan="3">Clarification of training needs</td></tr>
<tr><td></td><td colspan="4">Transfer of knowledge and experience</td></tr>
<tr><td></td><td colspan="4">Retention of challenging jobs</td></tr>
</table>

Field of promotion	Physical strain	Psyche / cognition	Mental / social competence	Professional competence
	Promote new job areas for seniors			
	Active quest for senior employees			
Communication	Free consultancy for launching of senior policy initiatives			
	Significant influence of seniors on their workplace			
	Putting senior concerns and their conditions on the company's agenda			

** Exercise, nutrition, consumption of alcohol and nicotine, relaxation*

Fig. 4: Summary of actions - Denmark

1. Political basis

1.1. The Danish Ministry of Employment

The Danish Ministry of Employment is responsible for the joint strategy for all unemployed persons; i.e. both the recipients of cash benefits from individual and private insurances (in many cases part of trade union membership) and the recipients of benefits from the federal unemployment insurance. It is furthermore responsible for the rules and the framework of employment and working conditions, the working environment, and industrial injuries, for maintenance benefits to all unemployed persons who are fully or partly fit for work and for job placement, and for services to business. The Ministry of Employment has established the need to strengthen and develop political measures concerning senior citizens. This is because the future labour force will consist of fewer young and more ageing workers, and anyone becoming redundant in later life will have difficulty in finding a job.

This view also characterises the National Action Plan for Employment of 2004, in which there is reference to governmental initiatives for older members of the workforce. It includes political initiatives for senior citizens, such as the possibility of deferred state retirement benefits or advising companies on senior policy. At the same time it stresses that measures to promote and support social commitment in companies have proven successful and that these actions should continue to receive support in future. Social commitment also comprises health promotion for the workers, irrespective of age.

In conclusion, it is evident that both social commitment on the labour market and a policy for ageing workers are encouraged, but there is no direct link between the two policies. Rather, it seems that they apply to workers in general.

1.2. The Danish Ministry of the Interior and Health

The Ministry of the Interior and Health is responsible for tasks related to health policy, in terms of financing and organising the health service, the legal position of patients, and the rights and obligations of health care staff. Supervising the health service and the pharmaceutical and medical fields are among its other responsibilities, as are also the prevention of diseases, health promotion, and health service statistics and analyses. Further issues are the international collaboration in the health domain and the municipal and federal emergency management.

1.3. The Amalgamation of Local Government

In the ongoing amalgamation of local governments 271 municipalities will become about 100 new municipalities and 13 counties will become five new regions. Thus, the incorporation of the existing 15 Acts on Health into one single Act, i.e. the Health Act, has been launched. This new Act will assign the creation of a framework for healthy living to the municipalities while the newly created regions will be responsible for providing facilities for medical treatment.

2. National programmes / projects

2.1. A Lifetime of Good Health

"A Lifetime of Good Health - National Objectives and Strategies for Public Health 2002-2010" is aimed at a broad collaboration of all Danes to achieve better health. It is a general health programme built on significant objectives from earlier programmes. The overall purposes were kept: increasing life expectancy, improving quality of life and social equality in health, measures for a number of risk factors, target groups, and day care institutions, at schools, in the workplace, and in the health service. Risk factors were identified: nicotine and alcohol abuse, unbalanced nutrition and physical activities and the resulting severe overweight, as well as accidents, the working environment, and overall environmental factors. An important prerequisite for a targeted effort is finding an appropriated starting point within the respective groups, one of these being senior citizens.

2.2. The Self-activation Pool for Senior Networks

In the Finance Act, funds have been earmarked for self-activation initiatives for senior citizens, which are intended to help unemployed job-seeking citizens over 50 years to obtain ordinary employment. Funds are provided for networking activities such as job search, project development, clarification of training needs, transfer of knowledge and experience, and projects promoting a range of new jobs for senior citizens.

2.3. Senior Policy Advisory Services to Companies

The senior policy advisory services scheme offers free consultancy to companies concerning the launch of policy initiatives for ageing workers. The advisory services comprise consultation of up to five hours with well-informed experts paid by the Directorate General for Employment, Placement and Vocational Training. The companies are assisted in developing or adjusting an existing policy for elders, in the preparation of training and hiring policies, and in establishing a network for exchange of experience between companies. Target groups of the scheme are mainly small and medium-sized private enterprises and company networks, nevertheless public companies and non-profit organisations may use the scheme to some extent.

2.4. The Senior Pool

For several years now, funds have been earmarked in the Finance Act for the launching of new initiatives aiding unemployed senior citizens to become reemployed and to retain older workers on the labour market. Grants are given to public companies, to labour market organisations, to associations, and to public institutions that solve tasks related to the issue of ageing. In 2004, grants were given to a project on factors for best practice for the employment and integration of unemployed senior citizens, a senior scheme in eldercare including the preparation of individual health profiles, and also to a project concerning the need for personnel policy practices in small and medium-sized enterprises.

2.5. The Working Environment Council

The Working Environment Council monitors the development in working environments and raises the issues held significant for these environments. It presents its recommendations and views on the objectives and the coordination of the work of the authorities and parties involved to the Minister of Employment. An annual report to the ministry is prepared concerning the development in the working environment domain, including any improvements desired by the council. The overall plan and objective of the work of the council from 2004 to 2007 includes workplace health promotion.

3. Players

3.1. NGOs / interest group representatives

3.1.1. Danish Confederation of Trade Unions (LO)

The Danish Confederation of Trade Unions (LO) is very keen on helping its members - mainly unskilled and skilled workers - to stay on the labour market as long as possible. This is because it acknowledges that the labour force must be increased to ensure future welfare. An effective means of increasing the workforce is to raise the average retirement age. As a consequence, LO wants the qualities of older workers to be recognised and supports an active senior policy. Thus LO favours jobs for older citizens that are flexible in terms of working hours and tasks. LO also supports health policy initiatives at workplaces.

LO itself has launched a very big campaign on preparing people for the labour market who are at risk of being excluded. One element of this is to consider the individual's fitness for work; however, it is left to the individual workplace to solve the health policy tasks. There is no direct connection between the labour market, health policy, and policy for older workers, as - in LO's opinion - labour market policy and health policy should apply to all the employees at a given workplace.

3.1.2. DaneAge Association (Ældre sagen)

"DaneAge Association" is the largest lobby in Denmark organising older people. The association is active in improving conditions for older people, including health issues and matters related to the labour market. "DaneAge Association" works on obtaining flexible employment conditions for older workers, e.g. part-time employment, retention of challenging jobs with continuing opportunities, training, and upgrading. At the same time "DaneAge" seeks to ensure that older workers have a significant influence on their workplace. "DaneAge Association" also works on promoting a healthy lifestyle among older people by initiating courses, thematic days, and lectures on these subjects.

3.1.3. Danish Trade Union of Public Employees (Fag og arbejde - FOA)

Fag og arbejde (FOA), the Danish trade union of skilled and unskilled public employees, works to make policy on ageing workers an integral part of the personnel policy. This policy comprises:

- interviews for employees over 50 with the purpose of personal assessment and planning for the future,
- training and development of competences with the purpose of maintaining and developing the competences of older workers,
- job development, taking into account special skills which may be useful,
- decreased working hours and increased leisure time, including flexible working hours,
- policy on older workers and the working environment, including the prevention of physical degeneration, and considering the abilities of older workers, and
- individual schemes for older workers, including transfer to senior positions and reduced working hours.

Furthermore, tools have been developed to put individual topics on the agenda for negotiation between the management and the employees. The agreements on senior policy between the trade unions and the municipalities are only considered as a starting point. Individual agreements on a local basis can always go beyond these general deals.

An example is the agreement between Birkerød Municipality and the child-minders and their organisations (FOA), which include child minders from 55 years and above.

Child-minders take care of small children in their own homes. To get their full salary they have to take care of four children each. When child-minders turn 55 and have been employed for more than 10 years, they can apply to be a part of the senior programme which gives them the right to take care of one child less and still get the full salary.

At the moment, the programme includes two of the municipality's 36 child-minders.

3.2. Private / commercial service enterprises

3.2.1. COWI (Consultancy within Engineering, Environmental Science and Economics)

COWI is one of Denmark's largest consultancy firms performing health financial analyses, evaluation, technology assessment, work procedure analyses, quality control, and organisational development tasks in the health area. Among other things they contribute to the preparation of a working environment label covering accomplishments in the working environment, the standard of the working environment, social responsibility, health promotion, staff development, and the organisation of work in the company.

3.2.2. Discus

Discus is a private consultancy company specialising in human resources on the labour market, including the social responsibility and policy on seniors of the companies they advise. Among other things they prepared a large development project to change the policy on seniors and health promotion in eight large and medium-sized companies in the Aarhus area. The companies participating have initiated a number of different sub-projects. On the basis of experience from this project, an advisory tool for companies and employees has been developed containing ideas to improve and initiate senior policy measures in workplaces.

The advisory tool developed was not ready until January 2005, and this is why there are no significant experiences with this tool yet. However, there are experiences from the development project. The individual companies decided for themselves what they wanted to work with. Here are some examples:

- A survey was made on the employee's attitude to senior policies.
- Statistics were made on the age distribution of the employes.
- Initiatives were taken to put seniors and their working conditions on the political agenda of the companies.
- Courses were provided to inform older workers about the conditions of retirement before they actually retired.
- Special employment contracts for seniors who wanted to reduce working time were made; existing agreements were

considered as well as the possibility of early retirement scheme or future pensions etc.
- Tools to structure the debate on senior policy in companies' works committees were generated.

3.2.3. Authorised occupational health services

Under Danish law, the National Labour Inspection may make it mandatory for Danish companies to seek advice if screening indicates that the working environment is not up to standard. Most of this advice is provided by a large number of working environment consultancy companies - so-called occupational health services - that used to be associations with statutory members. These companies have a great amount of specialised knowledge and experience in health promotion, advising on ergonomic workplace development and the like.

3.3. Research organisations

3.3.1. National Institute of Occupational Health

The National Institute of Occupational Health is a research institute within the public sector under the Ministry of Employment. It must contribute to creating a safe working environment which develops in accordance with the technical and social advances in society. The National Institute of Occupational Health is also a national centre for working environment research. The institute is concerned with strategic research and contributes to securing the widest possible coordination of Danish working environment research.

4. Projects

4.1. Industry

4.1.1. LM Glasfiber

LM Glasfiber produces windmills and employs a global workforce of 2,500. The factory at Lunderskov in Denmark has about 270 employees. Responsibility, initiative, and forward thinking are the three core values that run through the company. The company believes that older workers show responsibility and are able to take initiative on their own. Moreover, older people have life experience, good listening skills, and greater patience than younger people.

The 270 employees are distributed in two factories - one produces wings and the other components. The occupational health service assists in improving the workplaces, but nevertheless, building the wing of a windmill is hard work. The senior workers may not be as fast as they used to be but they have the overview and the competence regarding the way a wing is moulded. If the older workers wish so, they may be transferred from the production to the component department, which is less physically demanding, but requires the ability to work independently and to meet the deadlines.

4.2. Trade

4.2.1. The Netto Chain

Dansk Supermarked Gruppen has more than 29,000 employees in Denmark and consists of several retail chains. One division is the Netto convenience store chain with 360 shops in Denmark alone. The recruitment policy of Netto emphasises that employees of every age are needed.

Netto has established four senior shops across the country. The shop most recently established is the senior shop at Udbyhøjvej at Randers, Denmark. Here, in collaboration with the employment agency, the chain recruited unemployed workers over 50 who were ready for a career shift and who had the right profile for working in a convenience store. The response was tremendous, and up to now 50 % of the shop employees are over 50 years old. The qualities of older workers emphasised are that they are seldom absent due to sickness, they match the customer group and they are independent, brave, and enthusiastic. In order to attract and retain older workers, the age distribution is as important as the fact that older workers are directly targeted. The existence of a written senior policy including various health promotion activities is just as relevant.

4.3. Social services

4.3.1. Holbæk Municipality

The central administration at Holbæk Municipality employs a staff of more than 280 and has a value-based personnel policy, which just states that the municipality wants to retain its senior employees. However, the policy includes eight values and corresponding norms concerning objectives and measures, which makes the municipality an attractive employer. Although the municipality wishes to retain its senior workers it makes no special offers to them. However, other objectives and measures in the personnel policy, such as a good working environment and working climate, contribute to encouraging older workers to stay longer. An active effort is also made with health promotion and this also contributes to retaining older workers.

4.3.2. Storstrøm County Psychiatric Services

Storstrøm County Psychiatric Services, which has over 1,250 employees, have launched a project with the general purpose of postponing the retirement age by at least one year in comparison to now. The following two issues are being discussed: what values and perspectives senior workers have in relation to their work and whether the jobs held by seniors comply with these values.

Based on the outcome of the survey, the psychiatric services want to propose the use of personnel policy tools which ensure that work is worthwhile - especially for senior workers. In contrast to the most common approach when considering senior workers, this project takes an individual stance. Instead of considering senior employees as a fairly homogeneous group sharing the same beliefs and values - irrespective of the group's composition otherwise - the starting point of action here is focused on frequent age-related problems such as reduced health and lack of speed.

4.4. Services

4.4.1. Knuthenborg Safari Park

Knuthenborg Safari Park is a zoological garden employing 75 permanent and 75 seasonal workers with an even distribution of men and women. Many of the seasonal workers are young students, thus older workers have to be actively recruited to secure a reasonable age distribution among the staff.

The jobs are adjusted to the individual employees. The development of a good physical and psychological working environment has been initiated - including health promotion for all employees. Flexible working hours are an option.

Finland

Riitta-Maija Hämäläinen

<table>
<tr><th>Field of promotion</th><th>Physical strain</th><th>Psyche / cognition</th><th>Mental / social competence</th><th>Professional competence</th></tr>
<tr><td>Action</td><td colspan="4"></td></tr>
<tr><td>Relief of physical strain / WHP actions</td><td colspan="2">Setting-based actions</td><td></td><td></td></tr>
<tr><td></td><td colspan="2">Behaviour-based actions *</td><td></td><td></td></tr>
<tr><td></td><td colspan="3">Reducing / balancing of physical work-load of ageing operators without loss in salary</td><td></td></tr>
<tr><td></td><td colspan="4">Participatory ergonomic development</td></tr>
<tr><td></td><td colspan="3">Promotion and maintainance of physical exercises</td><td></td></tr>
<tr><td></td><td colspan="4">Mentorship</td></tr>
<tr><td>Age-related working hours</td><td colspan="2">Part-time pension</td><td></td><td></td></tr>
<tr><td></td><td colspan="3">Flexible working time arrangements / renovation of working times</td><td></td></tr>
<tr><td></td><td colspan="3">Part-time leave from work</td><td></td></tr>
<tr><td></td><td colspan="3">Sabbatical leave as regular possibility</td><td></td></tr>
<tr><td></td><td colspan="3">Rescheduling / reducing three-shift working systems</td><td></td></tr>
<tr><td></td><td colspan="3">Regular and quick rotation in shifts</td><td></td></tr>
<tr><td></td><td colspan="3">Micro-breaks</td><td></td></tr>
<tr><td>Qualification</td><td colspan="4">Lifelong learning (support training without limitations)</td></tr>
<tr><td></td><td colspan="4">Expanding supply of open learning environments (distance secondary school, Open University etc.)</td></tr>
</table>

Field of promotion	Physical strain	Psyche / cognition	Mental / social competence	Professional competence
	Increasing multi-skilled workforce and teamwork			
	Training of leadership skills			
	Improving / adopting of supervisory and management practices			
	Transfer of tacid knowledge			
Communication	Development of reward systems			
	Change attitude of employers and employees towards respecting the aged			
	Democratic dialogue between employers and employees			
	Development of a work ability index			
	Interest monitoring by trade unions and employer's organisations			
	Intensified cooperation of all parties involved in workplace development			
	Lobbying in relation to ageing at work by stakeholders			
	Building company networks (related to different industries and within and between regions)			
	Creating specific "Ageing and Work" pages on the WorldWideWeb			
	Producing promotion materials (guides, videos, tv/radio series, articles, seminars etc.)			

** Exercise, nutrition, consumption of alcohol and nicotine, relaxation*

Fig. 5: Summary of actions - Finland

1. Prerequisites

1.1. Definition of workplace health promotion in Finland

For the term workplace health promotion an equivalent term in Finland is the maintenance and promotion of work ability (TYKY-toiminta in Finnish). The maintenance and promotion of work ability at workplaces includes "activities aiming at maintaining the ability to work including all measures taken by the employer and the employees, as well as the cooperative organisations at the workplace, in a united effort to promote and support the ability to work, and to enhance the functional capacity of all persons active in working life throughout their working careers".

The Collective Agreement between employers' associations and trade unions, in which promotion and maintenance of work ability was defined, was agreed in 1989. The promotion and maintenance of work ability as the employers' obligation was included in the Occupational Health Service Act in 1991.

Targets of WHP are presented in the below Figure 1. Workplace Health Promotion supports the well-being and functional capacity of employees, and advances workplace functions and productivity.

The central factors (quality criteria) in Workplace Health Promotion are, that work ability is a broad and many-sided concept. WHP requires participation of the management and personnel as genuine and direct partner. WHP needs resources for the activities, which are based on the requirements of the workplace. The successful process of development of WHP at workplace is cooperative and applies to everyone at the workplace. In addition, the process is continuous, goal-oriented, planned and documented at the organisational level. For the continuous improvement of WHP follow-up, evaluation and corrective measures are made (http://www.tyky.fi).

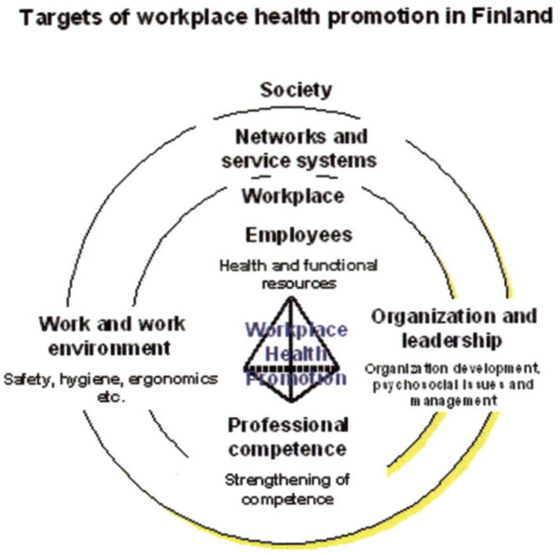

Figure 6: Maintenance and promotion of work ability in Finland (Ilmarinen et al. 1995)

1.2. Political basis

The Collective Agreement between employers' associations and trade unions was agreed in 1989. The promotion and maintenance of work ability was included into the Occupational Health Service Act in 1991 as an obligation for the employer.

The Council of State set up a Committee to chart the prerequisites for employing ageing (45-55-year old) and older (55-65-year old) persons. The Committee introduced 40 recommendations. The Council of State made a decision in principle for the National Programme on Ageing Workers in 1997 for the years 1998-2002 to put the recommendations into practice with the slogan "experience is a national treasure".

During the Presidency of EU in 1999, Finland focused on the ageing workforce and their work ability and gained significant support in the EU. Two important publications were produced, one on ageing workers in EU and a report on the action programme to promote the health, work ability and well-being of ageing workers (Ilmarinen 1999, Ilmarinen, Louhevaara 1999).

The strategy of the Ministry of Social Affairs and Health for social and health policies supports workplace health promotion through the occupational health services, in cooperation with work, the work environment, employers, and employees, in order to help prolong working life and to increase work ability. The strategy underlines well-being at work, and health and safety in working conditions.

The Ministry of Labour aims to raise the employment rate among the ageing work force in the age groups (55-64) by the year 2010 up to 50 %. The national aim is to raise the retirement age by three years, which would mean that the employment rate would be over 60 %. There are several measures the ministry will take to achieve these aims. Since 1992, the ministry has published annually a working life barometer which also includes topics related to work ability.

2. National programmes / projects

2.1. Respect for the Ageing (FinnAge)

This action programme was carried out from 1990-96 and was aimed at promoting the health, work ability and well-being of ageing workers. After conducting several case studies, models of good practice were created and tested in a broad-based cooperation within companies and organisations. Supporting the work ability of ageing workers was done by a combination of measures with the aim of having a positive affect on the work environment, the work organisation and the individual worker. The Finnish Institute of Occupational Health, in collaboration with several universities in Finland, was in charge of the programme (Ilmarinen, Louhevaara 1999).

The models of good practice were given as handbooks: "Work Ability and Welfare from Exercise: Principles and Examples from Practice", "Good Work Ability: Maintenance Handbook for Work Ability", and "A Handbook on Ageing and Work".

The measures, which affect the work environment, work organisation and the individual workers, were tested in industry, the public sector and municipalities. In industry the main sectors were the metal, construction and clothing industries. Strategies used were: changing the attitude of employers and employees to respect ageing, rescheduling three-shift systems, reducing the physical work-load of ageing operators, improving cooperation between different generations of workers (e.g. between young and old), promoting physical exercise, job redesign (teamwork, participation on job design) and the development of a work ability index.

In the public sector the major occupational groups were fire-fighters, police officers, vehicle inspectors, professional cleaners and teachers. The measures used were among others evaluation of job demands and work, and mental, physical and health capacities for work. In addition measures for improved ergonomics and work load reduction were developed.

In the municipal sector the major groups for maintenance and improvement of work ability were ageing home care workers, pipe and rail fitters, health care workers and municipal workers. Measures developed included improvement of ergonomics, support to physical exercise and other lifestyle determinants, balancing of physical work load, treatment of low back pain, improved shift work and computerisation taking into consideration the workers' occupation and age (different training approaches for ageing workers with low computer skills).

2.2. Research Programme on Ageing

The Research Programme on Ageing ran from 2000-2002 at the University of Jyväskylä. The main task was the production of information to help in dealing with problems and challenges associated with the ageing of workforces. It was expected that information for practical application in various sectors would be generated. The research issues spread over housing and employment, health policy planning and treatment methods. At the same time it was intended to increase the involvement of the academic research community in the ongoing public debate on ageing. The programme consisted of 21 projects from 12 universities and institutes involving over 100 researchers. Funding was provided by the Academy of Finland. (http://www.uta.fi/laitokset/tsph/itu)

Of special interest were the following research projects in the Research Programme on Ageing:

a) The Labour Market Challenge of Workforce Ageing (The Research Institute of the Finnish Economy - ETLA)

The project contributed to the understanding of how the Finnish labour market has so far adapted to workforce ageing. By means of in-depth micro-level analyses of the restructuring, functioning and capacity of the Finnish labour market, potential problems impairing successful integration of the ageing workforce were detected and, consequently, pointed to policies that were expected to enhance this process.

The project approached the challenges of workforce ageing from the demand side, the supply side, and pension and social security policies. The demand-side analysis focused on the changing skill requirements and demand for heterogeneous labour and the consequences for the recruitment of and relative demand for ageing workers. The supply-side analysis highlighted the employment, earnings and mobility of ageing workers. The public policy analysis explored the impact of changes in pension and social security programmes. Linking these highly interrelated domains produced a more complete picture of the labour market situation in Finland of ageing workers than provided in previous studies.

b) Health, Functioning and Well-being among Ageing Employees - The Helsinki Health Study (University of Helsinki; Department of Public Health)

The main aim of the Helsinki Health Study was to examine the impact of biological, psychosocial, behavioural, work related and socio-economic factors on health, functioning and well-being among ageing employees. Attention was given both to determinants promoting health and those producing ill-health, by (amongst other methods) simultaneously studying the effects of work and home characteristics on health; identifying the most pertinent dimensions of socio-economic position on health, and examining the causes of socio-economic inequalities in health; establishing the causes of health and functioning decline, sickness absence and early retirement among ageing employees. Data was collected from women and men aged 40+. The data combined questionnaires, registers and medical examinations. Determinants and health outcomes included health behaviours, anthropometric measurements, biological risk factors, general health and illness, mental and physical functioning, well-being, major diseases and mortality.

2.3. The National Programme on Ageing Workers

This programme was implemented from 1998 to 2002 using legislative and educational approaches, a media campaign, and research and development resources. The programme focused on research, training and dissemination of information to reform working life structures. The objective of the programme was to strengthen the status of ageing persons on the labour market as well as to improve their chances of staying at work, and to help them to find employment. Instead of concentrating on maintaining the physical working capacity as before, the emphasis now was on mental coping, individuality, flexibility, methods of management, and discussions as a means of interaction.

Within the Programme on Ageing Workers the information about the use of part-time pension was intensified. From the beginning of June 1998, it was possible to retire on a part-time pension at the age of 56, instead of 58, as it was previously. Another part of the programme was to examine whether the employers' contribution for disability pensions could be reduced.

Flexible working time arrangements and measures to develop work communities were also identified as important for the employment of ageing persons and maintaining their working capacity. Their training is to be improved by experimenting with methods combining working life and the training of ageing employees. The expanding supply of open learning environments (distance secondary school, Open University, networks of liberal education) facilitates the access of employed adults to education and training. Another objective of the projects was to improve working life to promote the interaction between employees of different ages at workplaces.

The programme was based on the proposals of the committee surveying the prerequisites for employing ageing (45-55) and older (55-65) persons. When the decision was taken to launch the programme, legislative amendments were also decided upon. A new paragraph was added to the Act on Codetermination in Companies: "Personnel and training plans should seek to devote attention to the special needs of ageing workers and officials". Amendments were made to the Occupational Safety Act; ageing was added to the list of issues that employers must take into account in addition to age, gender, vocational skills etc. Also workplace health promotion was added to the programme, i.e. employers are required to promote safety and health in the workplace. During the programme period of the National Programme on

Ageing Workers, a new Occupational Health Care Act was enforced (beginning in 2002). The main responsibility for the programme was borne by the Ministry of Social Affairs and Health; other responsible parties were the Ministry of Labour and the Ministry of Education.
(http://pre20031103.stm.fi/suomi/ikaohjelma1998-2002/)

2.4. The Well-Being at Work Programme

From 2000 to 2003, the programme focused on research, development and information dissemination. It aimed to promote working capacity and competence, and to help to maintain well-being at work. The motivation for the programme lay in alterations in working life mainly caused by changes in the external working environment. Employees are expected to learn new skills, and the willingness and ability to deal with this constant learning have become essential.

The Ministry of Labour and the Ministry of Social Affairs and Health were responsible for the project implementation, together with the Ministry of Education, the Ministry of Trade and Industry, the labour market organisations, and other stakeholders. Representatives of entrepreneurs, agricultural producers, sports organisations, and the Church were also involved in the programme.

Within the programme the tendency of Finns to leave the labour market at a relatively early age was addressed. The challenges of demographic change and the high stress levels revealed by work climate studies were also issues in the programme.

The target groups for the programme consisted of a broad range of companies, public bodies, organisations, entrepreneurs, and farmers. In addition to ageing workers' well-being at work, the programme also focused on young adults. It operated on four levels: the provision of information and dissemination of good practices, the utilisation of existing research findings and initiation of new research, support for development projects, and monitoring of legislation work.

The evaluation report showed that the key value added by the Well-Being at Work Programme was that it increased awareness generally through its extensive information provision and dissemination of good practices. Well-being at work is the result of the combined effect of several factors. The programme emphasised supervisory and management practices and interaction, people's control over and mastery of their own work, the transfer of tacit knowledge, the organisation of work, and working time arrangements, which can also help people coordinate family life and work.

The research projects within the programme also clearly demonstrated that well-being at work is not a mere coincidence or the result of isolated actions, but requires determined, systematic development work. One of the new research results is the fact that the health and well-being of staff are part of an organisation's intellectual capital. This is forgotten in most surveys on intellectual capital.

The development projects highlighted the need for day-to-day management, learning-on-the-job, and arrangements for working times and methods. Successful development projects were characterised by the following: cooperative and interactive development, good leadership, and trust and openness.

A study of working hours arrangements showed that at workplace level working time must answer the needs of the company or organisation as well as those of its employees in a balanced fashion. Management of working time emerged as a crucial factor in the prevention of exhaustion and burnout.

Combination indicators based on personnel strategy secure the planning, steering and monitoring of an organisation. The empirical material brought forth results that are significant with regard to economy: personnel satisfaction correlates significantly with client satisfaction. The same correlation appears in large-scale enterprises between personnel satisfaction and management and the upgrading of skill. (http://www.mol.fi/jaksamisohjelma)

2.5. The Finnish National Workplace Development Programme

The Finnish National Workplace Development Programme (1996-99, 2000-03) aimed to boost productivity and the quality of work life by furthering the full use and development of staff know-how and innovative power at Finnish workplaces. The programme aimed at this by developing human resources and helping work organisations to reform their modes of operation. The research-assisted development programme supported workplace-initiated projects, sped up initiatives at the level of the workplace, boosted the use of research in developing working life, created and maintained cooperation networks to disseminate and built up knowledge and competence, and increased international information exchange. The programme supported projects set up on the initiative of companies and public-sector organisations. The areas in focus were among others promoting new forms of working and work organisation, developing management and cooperation skills, developing human resources with the specific target of increasing staff expertise and innovation, promoting the status of ageing people and young workforce as well as the interaction of workforce of various ages, and promoting gender equality. The programme was led by the Ministry of Labour in cooperation with the representatives of the central labour market organisations, the Confederation of Private Entrepreneurs and the Working Environment Division and the Occupational Safety and Health Division of the Ministry of Social Affairs and Health. (http://www.mol.fi/tyke/1996-99)

The second phase of the Finnish National Workplace Development Programme 2000-2003 aimed to promote effectiveness and the quality of work life by furthering innovation-supporting modes of operation and employee skills at Finnish workplaces. The main methods were to provide financial and other support and expertise for development projects at Finnish workplaces, to disseminate information and expertise on workplace development, and to intensify cooperation between all parties involved in workplace development.

Development projects typically focused on promoting team work and empowering methods of management, increasing multi-skilled workforce, improving coping at work and building networks between companies. Both managements and employees took part in planning and carrying out the projects. Two-thirds of the projects were carried out in the private sector, most of them in the manufacturing industry. Local authorities also took part actively in the programme. (http://www.mol.fi/tyke)

New forms of working and work organisations can be typified as skill development based on the company's vision and strategy to improve work ability and competitiveness of the company - aimed at defining key competences and needs of competences, improving management, and supporting learning as a value and company culture. Other new forms were development of order-manufacturing processes towards a self-directing factory, democratic dialogue between employers and employees and development of regional networks between related industries. Installation of multi-skilled and team work as well as improving productivity through consultancies and mentorship, interaction and cooperation skill development, physical activities, and evaluation and promotion of work ability served as examples of new forms of work and work organisations.

2.6. National Productivity Programme

The programme was launched by the Economic Council in 2000, and ran until 2003. The main objectives were to improve the functioning of work communities, to speed up productivity improvement in companies and organisations, to promote the competitive edge on international markets and to raise the employment rate and level of income. The research projects aimed at creating changes in work practices and modes of operation and promoting the well-being of employees, as well as improving productivity. The priorities recorded were to improve and utilise the competence of employees at various stages of their career by developing the work organisation and workplace culture, to develop suitable methods and practices for improving the productivity of SMEs in the industrial and service sectors, and to launch development projects related to the application of know-how related to productivity. The National Productivity Programme was a follow-up of the programmes implemented in 1996-1999 (The Productivity Programme) and 1993-1995 (The Productivity for the Future Campaign). The labour market organisations, the government, the municipalities and numerous entrepreneurs stood behind the programme. (http://www.tuottavuus.net)

The research projects produced a lot of suggestions to improve the quality of workplaces and productivity, such as the following: increase productivity through monitoring, define industry-specific measures and indicators and flexibility of tasks, production or work environment.

The development of quality standards for work environment were initiated by use of total quality management and balanced scorecards at workplaces. As a key measure was addressed the development of networks between industries and within industries. A rise in productivity was achieved through the empowerment of workers, integration of productivity and safety at work and through changing organisational structures (more team work, project management, participatory management, joint consultancy, risk management etc.). Knowledge sharing and value reproduction in knowledge work and development of reward systems etc. were key issues for attaining better performance at work.

2.7. The National Action Programme for Prolonging Working Life, Employee Well-being and Rehabilitation (VETO - www.vetoatyoelamaan.fi)

This national action programme started in 2003, and will run until 2007. It focuses on developing the activities of institutions, such as occupational safety and health inspectorates, occupational health service providers, and rehabilitation institutes, which help workplaces to cope with the issues mentioned. The programme deals with factors that influence the maintenance and promotion of an individual's ability to work, prevention of marginalisation from work life, prevention of premature incapacity to work, and improvement of opportunities to return to work. The main responsibility for the programme is within the Ministry of Social Affairs and Health. Other participants in the programme are the labour market organisations, entrepreneurs' organisations, Ministry of Education, Ministry of Labour, Ministry of Trade and Industry, and the Finnish Institute of Occupational Health. The programme continues on the same issues developed in earlier programmes, such as the National Programme for Ageing Workers and the National Well-being at Work Programme. www.stm.fi

Work ability will be promoted and maintained through prevention of musculo-skeletal diseases by new ergonomics and also methods to be developed for specific professions prone to lifting and repetitive strains. Improving mental well-being at work, support for those wanting to stay on at work, and the prevention of occupational injuries and diseases will help to maintain and promote work ability.

Mental well-being will be promoted through materials prepared in previous programmes. Furthermore, information and training, creating an encouraging work environment, improving control over work and decreasing violence and mobbing at work will promote mental well-being at the workplace. The target groups are ageing workers and their "survival" in demanding or high workload situations. The high number of ageing workers at work will require advice, consultation, information, and training at workplaces. Concerning the prevention of occupational injuries and diseases, the focus will be on the construction, industrial and transportation sectors, especially on young male workers.

The programme aims to improve employers' and employees' skills and practices in matters of health and safety through better information, motivation and improved skills. Safety management systems and tools for risk and work load management will be developed and distributed.

2.8. The Programme "Improve the Employability, Career Prospects and Length of Work among the Least Educated Adults" (NOSTE - www.noste-ohjelma.fi)

This programme also kicked off in 2000 and will run until 2007. It encourages the improvement of employee and entrepreneurial skills. In addition, the Ministry of Labour supports the training of unemployed, less skilled people so they can attain a professional examination or degree, as well as training in computer literacy, also for ageing people. Both the Ministry of Education and the Ministry of Labour are involved.

2.9. The Workplace Development Programme for the Improvement of Productivity and the Quality of Working Life (TYKES - www.tykes.fi)

This programme started in 2004, and will finish in 2009. The programme was included in the Government Programme and focuses directly on funding development activities at workplaces. The programme promotes new work and human resource management practices, and develops methods, models and tools tried out in programme-funded development projects. The programme should become a source of learning and inspiration for other workplaces and stakeholder groups as well. The management group appointed by the Economic Council of the Government comprises representatives from the government, the labour market organisations, the trade associations, and the sponsors of work life research. The programme is implemented by the Ministry of Labour jointly with the labour market organisations, the trade associations and other ministries (Ministry of Social Affairs and Health and Ministry of Trade and Industry).

The practices, methods and tools will be developed during the course of the programme. However, business processes, organisation and human resource development will be more integrated. This concerns also quality improvement processes, the maintenance of health and safety at work, workplace health promotion, and training issues. All these areas need improved coordination and connections to operational management. Other areas of improvement are the development of consultant based dialogues between professionals and position related groups (bottom-up, bottom-down) and a participatory approach to improve the participation of all concerned, through ideas, skills and knowledge of business development. Another area of improvement is the implementation of a company strategy with participatory methods such as improved communication and toolbox.

Significant sponsors of projects and programmes for development of Finnish work life:

1. The Finnish Work Environment Fund (TSR) was established in 1979, with the aim to improve the work environment, work life and productivity by funding research and the development and dissemination of information. The TSR provides substantial funding for several shorter and smaller development and research projects related to the ageing workforce. www.tsr.fi
2. The European Social Fund (ESF) engages in various activities for workplace development, like support for employment and lifelong learning, promotion of employment and social inclusion, and equality. The goals of the programme are, for example, equal treatment at work, to improve the quality and impact of training, prolonging working life, and renovating work life. Objective 3 of the ESF Programme and the EQUAL Community Initiative are the most important ones. In the case of Objective 3 of the ESF Programme project funding takes place at a regional level and in the EQUAL Community Initiative at a national level (www.mol.fi, 7.10.2004). ESF is one of the largest funding sources for workplace development projects at regional and national level. ESF Objective 4 Programme for the Employed aids SMEs in improving their efficiency and ability to cope with new market challenges, in which Finland has included the maintenance of work ability or workplace health promotion.

About a hundred projects were started under the umbrella of ESF part-funding (Liira J., Rasanen M-L. 2001).

3. Players

3.1. NGOs / interest group representatives

3.1.1. Trade Unions

3.1.1.1. Local Authority Employers (KTV - www.ktv.fi)

KTV primarily influences legislation, e.g. most recently employees' training and education in relation to competence requirements, tasks at work, task dimensions and possibilities for use, and improving skills at work. In addition, KTV offers services on quality improvement of working conditions to municipalities to improve the employees' well-being, including ageing workers. KTV supports professional development through courses and seminars, and gives financial support to such initiatives at workplaces. KTV conducts surveys and research projects to support work life among the ageing population. KTV participates in national programmes, such as NOSTE (see 2.8.) and TYKES (see 2.9.) as a member of the boards.

3.1.1.2. The Finnish Confederation of Salaried Employees (STTK - www.sttk.fi)

STTK has been involved in the process of amending legislation (e.g. Act on Work Contract, Act on Occupational Health Services, Acts on Pensions) in several committees. Through its sector trade unions, STTK has been involved in the development of work life. In the process of changing the Act on Pensions, STTK emphasised the individual transition phase to retirement, the possibility to lighten the work load without any impact on salary, and a part-time pension. STTK also supports sabbatical leave as a regular possibility. In centralised labour market settlements in 2004, the emphasis was on safeguarding social benefits in the phase of restructuring companies. STTK aims to develop joint action at work places to integrate employees and their representatives better to workplace improvement processes through joint recommendations and tools prepared by the employer and employee organisations.

The joint recommendations include a "Non-violence at Work" package and "Mirror of the Workplace" with criteria for a good workplace, and related materials to be used at workplaces.

3.1.1.3. Central Organisation of Finnish Trade Unions (SAK - www.sak.fi)

The aim of SAK is to underline ageing at work in centralised labour market settlements, especially in relation to working time and shift work. The work should be adapted to the age of the worker, and discrimination by age must not be allowed. SAK has emphasised that the ageing of workers and their well-being needs special attention. Several sector unions have included well-being at work in relation to older workers in the labour market contracts. The sector unions organise training on well-being at work and equality at work, but SAK rather emphasises the entire work life and the need to improve it. The renewal of training schemes is also related to ageing, as not many programmes have been developed for workers over 50 years of age, despite the increasing requirements to lengthen the work career. In addition, SAK favours long-term contracts, and conducts interest monitoring and lobbying in relation to ageing at work and the government budget or legislation, for example.

SAK initiated a programme for national well-being at work, which was taken up by the government. In addition, SAK is involved in VETO (see 2.7.), NOSTE (see 2.8.) and TYKES (see 2.9.) programmes as a board member of the programmes.

3.1.1.4. The Confederation of Unions for Academic Professionals in Finland (AKAVA - www.akava.fi)

AKAVA aims to develop the quality of work life through part-time pensions to improve well-being at work. AKAVA is also involved in VETO (see 2.7.), TYKES (see 2.9.) and NOSTE (see 2.8.) programmes, and the member unions get information concerning these funding and project possibilities through AKAVA. In their training, ageing at work is related more to the improvement of the quality of work life in general than to separate issues. In addition, AKAVA promotes sabbatical leave as a permanent possibility; promotes a renovation of working times; supports training without limitation, and follows up several initiatives on equal treatment at work.

3.1.2. Employers' Organisations: The Confederation of Finnish Industries (EK; beginning with January 1, 2005 - www.ek.fi)

EK has emerged from the Employers' Confederation of Service Industries and the Confederation of Finnish Industry and Employers. The confederations have ad hoc training sessions on ageing at work. Otherwise the confederations are members of the boards of VETO (see 2.7.), TYKES (see 2.9.) and NOSTE (see 2.8.) programmes.

3.2. Private / commercial service enterprises

There are 123 units for research, development and training on work life issues. These include universities, centres for further training, polytechnic institutes, adult education centres and schools, research institutions, technological centres, and the research and education centres of trade unions and employers' organisations. In addition, there are more than 700 private consultancy agencies. Ageing is related to equal treatment at work, among several other activities which these units provide to workplaces. The services are provided as paid services, training, consultation, ordered surveys or studies, and training places. The services are provided mostly to enterprises and the public sector, mostly at municipalities, and with some activities in the third sector. The funding comes from foundations, scholarships or trusts, like The Academy of Finland, Technological Development Centre, Work Environment Fund, European Social Fund, the ministries, the Social Insurance Institute, or county councils. Other funding sources are government and international organisations, like EU programmes and Nordic trusts (Ramstad E. 2001).

3.3. Research organisations

3.3.1. Finnish Institute of Occupational Health (www.ttl.fi)

The Finnish Institute of Occupational Health also conducts several long-term and regular research and survey projects on, e.g. the ageing workforce, like the National Barometer of Maintenance of Work Ability (1998, 2001), the National Follow-up System for Occupational Health Services (1993, 1996, 1998, 2001) and Work and Working Conditions in Finland (1997, 2000). One long-term research project is the "Follow-up of Ageing Municipal Employers since 1981". It is planned to conduct the next follow-up in 2006 (Tuomi 1997). The Institute has created specific Ageing and Work pages on the Internet at www.ikatyo.fi. These pages describe ageing and the related challenges and goals from the viewpoint of the individual, the company and society. The pages provide public access to reliable information on ageing and work.

The institute underlines behaviour-based as well as setting-based actions to improve workers' health. Concerning shift-work, several suggestions to relieve work-stress are given: shift work should be reduced; at least a quick and regular rotation in shifts should be implemented. Shifts should not exceed 8 hours, whereas recreation between shifts should at least add up to 11 hours with a weekend off during shift rotations. After night-shifts there should be at least two days off. Also suggested is an increase of micro-breaks between work tasks (2-3 minutes).

Training in leadership skills and increase of functional capacity through physical activity are considered to be important issues.

As part of the national VETO programme (see 2.7.), the Finnish Institute of Occupational Health manages the "Sustainable Work Career Development (KESTO) 2003-2007" project. It develops measures based on research findings which promote the work ability, increase the attractiveness of work life, and promote social inclusion. The KESTO programme will identify from a holistic point of view the measures needed to promote work ability through individual, company and society (national programmes on public health, alcohol and non-smoking campaigns) perspectives. Other such measures are the prevention of unemployment and staying on at work after retirement age (good work habits, adaptation of work to the workers needs, resources and skills, promotion of those characteristics which promote health and well-being at work, resources of primary health care and OHS). In addition, measures for early rehabilitation and return to work will be developed through part-time leave from work, cooperation between occupational health services, employers and rehabilitation providers, enhanced motivation, and improved ability to return to work. The objective is to improve the workers' health, and upgrade competence and motivation as well as to enhance the preconditions for work. The KESTO programme is implemented in two stages: work life research findings are collected and analysed, and - based on findings - suggestions are made concerning the most important measures for developing work life. www.ttl.fi/kesto

3.3.2. National Research and Development Centre for Welfare and Health (STAKES - www.stakes.fi)

STAKES carries out research and development work on the ageing workforce, e.g. among the personnel of the social and health services sector. Their well-being at work has an impact on the services provided. STAKES conducts surveys and uses registers for its research on work absenteeism in relation to psychosocial factors at work, service efficiency and productivity, and attitudes, knowledge, organisation of work and work load in relation to well-being at work. In addition, STAKES develops, together with municipalities, the skills of personnel in information technology and develops training and education approaches suitable for work situations with several partners. Also the activation of unemployed people through training and rehabilitation is developed by STAKES together with several other actors.

3.3.3. National Public Health Institute (www.ktl.fi)

Most health problems are related to work ability and the quality of life, which in turn are related to infectious diseases, health and cardiovascular disease, cancer, diabetes, asthma and allergies, musculo-skeletal disorders, mental health, and injuries and accidents. The KTL aims to prevent such conditions and to promote the health of all age groups including the ageing workforce. The KTL conducts annually a health behaviour monitoring survey to obtain information on the population's main lifestyles and their time trends (Terveys 2000 by Aromaa, Koskinen). These monitoring systems also provide information for the use of health policy decision-making, and can be used for evaluating specific health promotion campaigns and programmes. In addition, every fifth year, a Finnish nutrition surveillance, and every 10-15 years a population-based health survey is conducted, including issues concerning the ageing population.

3.3.4. The Universities

The Universities of Jyväskylä, Lapland, Turku, Tampere and Helsinki, The Technical University of Helsinki, The University of Arts and Design, and Statistics Finland conduct different types of research related to management and ageing, ergonomics and ageing, technology and ageing, changes at work and the labour market, social benefits in relation to ageing and work (pensions, retirement etc.).

3.3.5. The Finnish Centre for Pensions (ETK - www.etk.fi)

ETK conducts research on the social and economic effects of pensions. The studies evaluate the activities and development needs of the earnings-related pension scheme, and the effects of the reforms carried out. The aim of the studies is to provide information to serve the development of the pension scheme. The themes include pre-retirement pensions, changes in work life (entering the labour market, working conditions, breaks in work history, length of the work history, self-employed persons and their pensions, a flexible retirement age [Gould 1997]), social protection internationally, and national economy and pensions.

3.3.6. The Research Institute of the Finnish Economy (ETLA - www.etla.fi)

The research on labour markets that has been carried out at ETLA over the past decade covers a broad scope of labour market topics both at the microeconomic and the macroeconomic level. The topics covered in the institute's labour market research include wage bargaining, wage determination, unemployment, indirect labour costs, working hours, and internal labour markets. Labour force structures, employment creation and destruction, employability, and social exclusion are among the questions studied.

3.3.7. Social Insurance Institute (KELA - http://www.kela.fi/tutkimus)

The KELA conducts research activities in the area of pensions and the ageing workforce (Hytti 1998).

4. Projects

4.1. Respect for the Ageing - A Programme for Promoting the Health, Work Ability and Well-being of Workers over 45 Years of Age, 1990-1996.

The goal was the promotion of health, work ability and well-being of ageing workers. An attempt was also made to improve the quality and productivity of work by improving the resources of ageing workers. The maintaining of work ability during ageing focused on development of concepts and models in promoting work ability according to the Finnish definition of WHP, participatory ergonomic development, development of work organisations and promotion and maintenance of physical exercise for workers. The programme included about 25 projects, the description of which can be found in the publication of Ilmarinen and Louhevaara, 1999. The project was the responsibility of the Finnish Institute of Occupational Health in cooperation with the universities of Helsinki, Jyväskylä and Tampere, and the Tampere University of Technology. Funding was provided by the Finnish Work Environment Fund.

4.2. The ABB Mahis programme, 1994-1998.

The objective was to improve the workers' health, ability to work and the work environment, especially focusing on older workers. In the beginning, the health status, work ability, functional capacity and work load of the workers were measured. Feedback and ergonomic advice were given, further examinations were conducted, and exercise groups were started. A three-year follow-up produced significant improvement in the workers' perceived health status. The Mahis programme created a new way of looking at work ability measures from the enterprise's point of view. The work ability and well-being of the company's personnel became the core of the action and affected the investment in working conditions, the health of the work community, the functional capacity of workers, and their professional expertise. Work ability measures were integrated into the quality system, the business strategy and the company's mission. The programme was managed by occupational health personnel, personnel administration developers, and researchers. It was carried out in three projects: the Health Project (to improve the health of all employees), the Work Ability Project (to improve their physical and psychological health status) and the Work Community Project (to point out that the employee has an impact on the contents of his/her work and the psychosocial work environment).

4.3. The Prime-age Programme

This programme aimed at improving work ability and professional expertise of ageing workers in SMEs. Action models in SMEs in cooperation with the occupational health personnel of the company and regional adult education teachers were developed in 1997-2000. The SMEs received additional resources for their work ability activities during the programme: information and exchange of views in several seminars. Several other projects in SMEs in relation to work ability and skills have been conducted in different regions since the Prime-age Programme.

4.4. Promoting the employees' work ability in small and medium-sized enterprises as a part of the National Programme for Ageing Workers, 1998-2002.

The project aimed to promote the work ability of employees in small and medium-sized enterprises, namely industry, the service sector and arts and culture. The aim was to create good models at the workplaces for promoting and maintaining the work ability of employees. The emphasis was on ageing workers in order to prevent their early retirement and to encourage them to work until the statutory retirement age. The task of the project group was to support the start-up and implementation of the development work through discussions, meetings, interviews and consultations. Based on the start-up discussions, meetings, interviews, and consultations the enterprises often chose to implement training in vocational competence, as well as training in leadership skills. The older employees also participated in tailored training in information technology. The project was conducted by the Finnish Institute of Occupational Health.

4.5. Fitness for All Ages Action Programme, 1995-2000 and 2000-2004.

The objective was to increase the well-being, health and functional capacity of the ageing work force through physical activity. The methods were financial support, promotion and training to activate local projects. The specific criteria for the financial support were given and the best innovative approaches were awarded annually. The National Public Health Institute monitored the physical activity habits of the entire target group (40-60 years of age) as a part of health behaviour research. The action programme produced promotion material for the activities and the target group in the form of guides, videotapes, TV and radio series, newspaper and magazine articles, and training courses and seminars. The aim of the follow-up to the project was to find out what types of cooperative action produce good physical activity services and changes in living habits. http://www.kki.likes.fi

France

Marion Gilles, Michel Vallée

<table>
<tr><th>Field of promotion</th><th>Physical strain</th><th>Psyche / cognition</th><th>Mental / social competence</th><th>Professional competence</th></tr>
<tr><td>Action</td><td colspan="4"></td></tr>
<tr><td>Relief of physical strain / WHP actions</td><td colspan="2">Setting-based measures</td><td></td><td></td></tr>
<tr><td></td><td colspan="2">"Early retirement culture"</td><td></td><td></td></tr>
<tr><td>Age-related working hours</td><td colspan="2">Gradual reduction in working time</td><td></td><td></td></tr>
<tr><td>Qualification</td><td></td><td colspan="3">Integrated access to training courses</td></tr>
<tr><td></td><td colspan="4">Career management</td></tr>
<tr><td></td><td colspan="4">Adapted teaching methods for seniors</td></tr>
<tr><td></td><td></td><td colspan="3">Competence transfer between the generations / tutor scheme</td></tr>
<tr><td></td><td></td><td colspan="3">Motivation training till retirement</td></tr>
<tr><td>Communication</td><td colspan="4">Analysis of jobs and working conditions</td></tr>
<tr><td></td><td colspan="4">Survey of age structures</td></tr>
</table>

Fig. 7: Summary of actions - France

1. General context

1.1. Legislative context

In 1945, after WWII, a general retirement pension scheme was created in France based on the pay-as-you-go system, which confirmed the principle of retirement pensions for all.

Changes were made during the transition from 20th to 21st century: first in 1993 (the Balladur reform), which increased the contribution period for full pension entitlement in the private sector from 37.5 to 40 years, then in 2003, there was a pension reform increasing the period for contributions to 41 years by 2012 and 42 years by 2020.

In 1998, a reserve fund to preserve the pay-as-you-go system was established.

In France the ageing population is only seen in terms of pensions and the reforms necessary to uphold the pension system. There are differences between France and other countries regarding the national configuration of social protection and the chosen employment policies.

The French configuration can be summarised as follows[1]:

- Possible unemployment towards the end of working life is compensated for by a high level of social protection from the state, both in terms of amount and length of benefits.
- Because of this there is an almost total lack of integration instruments for older workers on the employment market.

This approach reflects the trend towards social transfer instead of keeping ageing workers at work longer. This trend to an "early retirement culture" means that French law has gradually shifted from protecting people against a loss of employment, as in the 1970s, to using age as the criterion to retire early. The "age-measures" which send older workers into early retirement widen the gap between those employees who benefit from reemployment programmes and those who don't.

Gradually, a definition of older workers emerges - they are at risk in their

[1] GUILLEMARD (Anne-Marie) "Societies dealing with ageing. The challenge of employment in the latter part of the career", in FUTURIBLES, n° 299, 08/2004.

occupation and unfit for reemployment. From this point of view it only seems fair to give easier access to social transfer to this segment of the population, so that soon the *right* of early retirement will be established. This is what is meant by forming an "early retirement culture" by making it easier for this group to access social transfer resources.

As generous public subsidies to encourage early retirement are widely accepted, attractive opportunities have been opened to both companies and employees at the expense of social transfer. Consequently job downsizing and mass unemployment have become the measures chosen to compensate whenever there is a slowdown in economic growth. The increase of unemployment in later life is an illustration of this policy. Furthermore, the rising number of unemployed young persons forced older workers to take advantage of age measures such as passive benefits without work. Older workers were asked to "make room for the young generation" by opting for pre-retirement status. Contrary to expectations, these measures had a disappointing effect on employment.

This process triggered a downgrading of older workers which will eventually affect even younger ones: the gap between "nearly-old" and "retirement agers" will widen and the position of "young" fifty-something or even forty-something workers on the labour market is weakened. Certain companies hesitate to promote or train them, as they are getting close to their "career end phase".

These facts generate a downward spiral that affects the whole latter part of their career - legitimate access to transfer resources for older employees has finally become an element that actively discourages the employment of older workers.

Employment rates for the 50-64-year-olds are low in France compared with other countries in the European Union. France was in the 9th position in Europe, with an employment rate of around 53 % in 2000. This rate has tended to increase over recent years because of the number of younger members of the 40-50 age group, with the fall off happening after the age of 55. In 2001, the employment rate was 85.7 % at 50 and 8.5 % at 64 years. The retirement rate is slow up to the age of 55, then very fast from 55 to 61 years.

So, if France would like to eliminate the "early retirement culture", there will have to be radical changes in the image of older employees as "unemployable", and measures to help workers to "grow old" in employment have to be found.

This, of course, cannot be done only by preventing access to early retirement by law or by reforming retirement regulations. A profound rethinking of the prevailing principles of social protection in France is necessary. Social protection should therefore move away from removing or compensating for risks at work and move toward new employment policies and improvements in human resource management.

For France, coping with an ageing workforce implies an unprecedented re-mobilisation in the employment of the 50-60 age group. A mobilisation effort on this scale has to be planned with an eye to medium- or long-term considerations. Keeping the 50-something age group in the employment market means having to maintain their employability, skills and competence. Also improving working conditions and building an organisation system adapted to the ageing of the workforce has to be done successfully. Finally, it will be necessary to design career structures that ensure the transfer of experience when there is a rapid renewal of generations at work. In France, these indispensable reforms are expected to be extraordinarily complex.

1.2. Political context[2]

1.2.1. Announced extension of working life: retirement pension reform, the Law of August 21, 2003

The law of August 21, 2003 - a retirement reform - aims at adapting the retirement system to the new financial and demographic structures. It will safeguard the pay-as-you-go system and relies principally on extending the required period of contribution for full pension entitlement.

Up to this day no active employment policy has yet been introduced to modify the status quo for older employees or to make them more attractive for employers. Therefore it is justified to ask if the intended extension of contribution periods will really result in a prolongation of active working life.

The fear is that sealing off some ways of early exit, like the progressive

[2] The French political context is very much in line with the objectives set by the European Union:
- In March 2001, the European Council of Stockholm aimed for an employment rate of 50 % for workers aged 55 to 64 by 2010,
- The Barcelona Council of March 2002, aimed for the gradual extension of the average retirement age by five years during the same period.

pre-retirement (PRP[3]) or ARPE, will lead to long-term ill health or invalidity within the group of older workers as a way to cope with their problems on the employment market. In that case money saved on retirement pensions may well be eaten away by benefits paid to those affected by long-term illness, invalidity or unemployment. This will be exacerbated if retirement systems are deprived of major financial margins - so far attained from the increasing age group of 50-60-year-olds. As young people entering the employment market will be less numerous and the rate of employment for women is already high in France, older persons will be the main reservoir of workers available in the forthcoming years.

1.2.2. Developing training throughout professional life: The national inter-professional agreement of September 20, 2003, concerning training throughout professional life

After three years of talks, the social partners agreed on a compromise that was signed by all of the negotiating parties. The entire *"Formation Continue"* professional training system (see 2.4.) has been completely overhauled, showing the determination of the social partners to adapt the training agreement system to the current situation in the world of work. In particular, the signatories have considered inequality of access to training and the demographic changes in France over the next 20 years. Employees aged 45 and over have been added to the target groups previously identified.

In detail, the agreement deals with professional training taking place under real working conditions and takes specific but not yet complete know-how into consideration.

1.2.3. Encouraging the employment of seniors

France has the lowest average retirement age in Europe. Up until the middle of the 1990s, employment policy consistently supported the withdrawal of seniors - i.e. 50-year-olds and up - from the employment market. Over the last ten years, the public authorities have strongly mobilised employment policy provisions to encourage a return to employment for seniors. Assisted employment is the principal approach chosen. It is used to ensure a profes-

[3] The PRP enables employees to shift to part-time work from the age of 55 and, as well as the part-time salary paid by the employer, receive a complementary allowance paid by the state. This system will be stopped at the end of 2004.

sional end to the working life of those becoming unemployed after what has often been a long career. Companies are exempt from charges in that programme and participants are not allowed to look for another job while they are on this programme.

However, the policy of withdrawal of employees over 50 years of age remains firmly anchored even though this age group qualifies for active employment measures. In reality, no new deployment has taken place between retirement policy (called "passive" policy) and policies encouraging elderly remaining in the employment market (called "active" policy).

2. Programmes and projects on national level or under study

In France, more than anything else, financing retirement pensions was the issue that drew public attention to the age and work concern.

2.1. Creation of COR: the Pensions Orientation Council

In 2000, the current government decided to create an authority in charge of advising on the problem of retirement pensions in the future. Certain reports submitted by this body focused on enlarging the debate on the development of the retirement pension system. They concentrated on the financial aspects of the problem, on the question of working conditions and on work plans that would enable working life to be extended effectively. The necessity of beginning negotiations between the social partners on the link between hardship at work and life expectancy was stressed.

After carrying out a study, the onus will be on the politicians to take the decisions according to their political orientation.

2.2. Report of the CES (Economic and Social Council): Age and Work in 2010

Commissioned by the Economic and Social Council (CES) the report presents a forecast of age management up to 2010. The report considers the upcoming demographic changes and reaffirms the need to upgrade the employment of employees in the "latter part of their careers". The author recommends that there should be a national think-tank process within companies for integrating access to training courses, career management, and the analysis of jobs and working conditions. The report addresses all players in charge of human resources management in companies, so that repercussions of these developments can be anticipated.

2.3. The COR Report: Difficulty and retirement

This report gives an inventory of current working conditions and different causes of hardship and difficulty at work. It presents and explains the correlation between difficult jobs and lower life expectancy, between difficult and dangerous jobs and between intricacy and tension at work. Hard and difficult working conditions have an impact on the period of contributions to be made for full rate pension eligibility. These relationships are being investigated further. Additionally, the COR stresses the necessity of negotiations between the social partners concerning this connection between physical workload and lowered life expectancy.

2.4. The Formation Continue (Professional Training) 2000 Report, by INSEE and CEREQ

The "Formation Continue 2000" surveys professional training use and its inequalities. Its indications led to a re-examination of public policy on encouraging professional training. In particular, this report examines the training methods and their use within companies. It raises the question whether training courses, as they are offered today, can help to retain any older person in employment. The analysis summarises a typology of the most common ways of running training courses. The issue is raised what content and teaching methods have to be developed for making the model of "training throughout life" effective.

3. Players

3.1. Institutions

3.1.1. The social partners

The social partners are fundamentally divided on the question of retirement. Not only is there disagreement between employers' and employees' representatives, but also amongst the employers themselves and between different trade unions. In the process leading to the new law on training throughout professional life (see 1.2.2), the government proposed that a framework should be negotiated by the social partners. An initial orientation was given by the government. This pre-project only found support within two union organisations.

Vocational training was also the subject of negotiations, which resulted in an agreement signed by all of the trade union organisations. Negotiation is required concerning the recognition of hardship and difficult work as a reason for modifying the contribution period for full retirement pension eligibility. However, the chaotic and conflict-ridden process has not yet resulted in any agreements.

3.1.2. ANACT (National Agency for the Improvement of Working Conditions)

ANACT is a public organisation belonging to the Employment Ministry and which consists of a tripartite board (state and the social partners). In the context of Progress Contract No. 3, signed by the state, the social partners and ANACT, the ANACT network is responsible for the development of the project of age management.

3.1.3. DARES (Research and Statistical Studies Executive)

Amongst other activities, DARES, a public structure, handles the ESSA survey (Employee jobs according to age), which focuses in particular on the ageing workforce and the way this is managed by companies. The survey's problem set can be summarised by the following questions:

- What is the structure per age group of employees?
- Is age an important criterion or even factor of discrimination in human resources management?

- How do companies perceive the demographic changes that are likely to affect them?
- Are they preparing to deal with this and, if so, what strategies do they intend to apply?

The mission and product of DARES is a regularly updated review of practices, approaches and collective mental attitudes towards ageing problems in working life providing information for all stakeholders.

3.1.4. AFPA (Adult Professional Training Association)

AFPA (http://www.afpa.fr/) is the main operator of the French Ministry of Social Affairs, Labour and Solidarity employing more than 10,000 staff members.

It develops a programme called "Work and Training at every Age", which tackles the specific features of learning according to age and professional experience and also recommends adapted teaching methods. Once again training on the job under actual working conditions is favoured, where specific but not yet complete know-how can be taken into account.

3.2. Business

3.2.1. Small to medium-sized businesses: the Agefos PME and IFOP survey of 1,000 companies, June 2004

While nearly 30 % of small to medium-sized and very small businesses will have to cope with workforce retirement over the next ten years, the perspective of an ageing working population is not one of their prominent preoccupations: only 7 % of very small businesses and 13 % of small to medium-sized businesses have set up specific means for dealing with this problem. Primarily, these actions focus on the organisation of competence transfer, dealing only slightly with the improvement of working conditions.

3.2.2. Are companies anticipating the ageing workforce? DARES, 2003

Managing the final part of the career remains the exception rather than the rule: in 2003, only one company head out of five admitted to using anticipative staff management according to age. It is more widespread in larger enterprises and in structures where the workforce in general is older. For enterprises of all sizes, "forward workforce management" is more frequently used with managerial staff, while when there is a high proportion of unskilled workers the opposite is true.

A well-known example of "forward workforce management" is Laboratoires BOIRON, the homeopathic market leader, where age management dates back to 1976, when there was an employee retirement preparation agreement.

The agreement consists of proposing a gradual reduction in working time, without any loss in salary, a maximum of six years before regular retirement age - compensatory allowances are given. This agreement allows a better balance between periods of work and periods of rest considering work difficulty and the age of the employee, forward staff planning, the transfer of competence between senior and junior staff with the introduction of a tutor scheme, and continuing motivation right up to the date of retirement.

3.3. Research

3.3.1. CREAPT (Working Population Age Research and Survey Centre)

Using a dual approach, both demographic and ergonomic, CREAPT's work deals with the overall problem of workforce ageing through statistical work, monographic analysis and surveys carried out in companies. It maintains a database of MOGP. (http://www.cee-recherche.fr/)

CREAPT suggests various degrees of individual freedom in organising working life according to age. Working conditions as well as work organisation must be suited to the modified abilities of different age groups. Considering the results of ergonomic studies, it suggests adapted and more "soft" work organisation.

3.3.2. CNRS (National Scientific Research Centre) and its Social Movement Study Centre

Numerous studies have been conducted on the ageing workforce; including comparative studies of European Union countries, the impact of ageing on human resources management, and on inter-generational cooperation. In particular, one study by Anne-Marie Guillemard gives the indication that social protection patterns and risk indemnities should act more in the field of "active policies" (i.e. policies encouraging elderly to remain in the employment market) than on rehabilitation measures. It also suggests considering a possible application of the Finnish National Employment Programme in France.

3.3.3. CEREQ (Employment and Qualifications Research and Study Centre)

CEREQ is particularly interested in the dynamics of careers, and provides a particular view into the process of exclusion from the employment market, linked with age.

In detail it demonstrates and develops an expulsion spiral from the labour market based on company selection patterns and the difficulty job-seekers have in formalising their experience and transferring it from one sector to another.

4. Projects

The ANACT network fulfils the needs of different organisations.

- Public institutions (Regional Councils, local authorities, government departments etc.) seek information on a macro level. They tend to aim at employment and training: demographic analysis of a local region, an employment area or particular sector, or prospective analysis of demography and employment, amongst others.
- The social partners will expect more specific input for different branches or professions. Their requirements also include methodology and evaluation tools for assessing hardship and difficulty, for example.
- Company interests are focused on retaining senior employees in their jobs as well as recruiting and integrating young employees.

There are two recurring questions in these demands:

- How to maintain good economic performance with a workforce that is often in a fragile state of health or lacks motivation?

- How to make the company more attractive for employees by integrating their different skills and competencies and providing them with a chance to gain experience?

The most concerns related to age management are about experience and work strain which can lead to deterioration in health. This means that, on the one hand, individual approaches taken by organisations towards "softer" working conditions and other actions for ergonomic relief are considered to be of overriding importance. However, on the other hand, collective approaches which reduce difficulties at work in general and collective agreements on regulations regarding these problems are also stressed.

4.1. Premature workforce fatigue prevention with Leroy-Somer

Leroy-Somer is one of the world's largest companies in the drive systems and alternators sector. The French factory at Gond-Pontouvre employs a workforce of 450 with an average age of 42 years. 39 % are aged between 50 and 60 years. Up until 2003, one of the responses to the ageing workforce was to use the early retirement system. Due to the demographic situation, production shifted to a continuous flow system with short production runs. But products have also become more complex and heavier, so multi-tasking had to be developed.

Training courses were set up to accompany these changes, as well as a system of professional trials to organise vocational development (work analysis, ergonomic approaches, sensitisation etc.). However, the current methods of managing ageing workers seem to have reached their limits, whether with the system of early retirement or the transfer of staff to "soft" posts.

Moreover, symptoms of "premature" ageing are appearing in younger generations, which are becoming more affected by the first signs of musculo-skeletal problems. Therefore the company now must face a double problem: managing employees over 55 and dealing with the premature appearance of symptoms of ageing amongst the younger generations.

To assist enterprises in their consideration of the problem, ARACT[4]

[4] Regional Association for the Improvement of Working Conditions

Poitou-Charentes, part of the ANACT network, carried out a preliminary training action analysing work with members of CHSCT (Comité d'hygiène, de sécurité et des conditions de travail - Commmittee on hygenie, security and working conditions), the occupational nursing office, occupational physician's office, heads of safety and methodology, and workshop supervisors in order to raise their awareness of the ergonomic approach. In a second phase, scenarios of organisational developments were worked out, based on the following criteria: employee health, production (deadlines, quality and volume), employment and cost. The freedom to organise work individually is possible when these criteria are considered.

4.2. A study of the difficulty of the refuse collector's activity for the SNAD (National Syndicate of Refuse Related Activities)

SNAD, the companies it represents, and its union leaders were interested in a study focusing on the work strains of its refuse collectors. For employees aged over 55 years the frequency and severity of accidents at work increases significantly. These facts made the branch study both the possibilities of early retirement for their employees and also ways to improve their working conditions. CREAPT and ANACT were given the responsibility for conducting such a study and submitting it to the joint steering committee in October 2003. Suggestions made were to reduce the workload by standardising refuse containers and to integrate health and security criteria in work specification. Also addressed was the possibility of changing careers.

Four types of data were used in highlighting the strain factors in the refuse collector's occupation: the analysis of data on the workforce and their state of health, interviews with retired refuse collectors, job observation, and analysis of the possibilities of a career structure.

4.3. Ageing and Job Difficulty: A Company Guide (In the framework of an EQUAL project)

Increased absenteeism, difficulty in managing the demands of multi-tasking because of reduced working ability, an increase in complaints from employees, the loss of know-how… In the absence of more precise indicators, age is often blamed for the problems companies are experiencing, yet it is often forgotten that the situation at work may be difficult for other age-groups too. ARACT Nord-Pas-de-Calais, part of the ANACT network, decided to help companies to approach the problem by using a more accurate diagnosis. ARACT drew up a guide showing the links between work strain and the age of workers. By cross referencing demographic indicators, data on working conditions and the health of employees, this guide enables companies to take action in their organisation. Twelve companies have already tested the guide.

In this way an initial diagnosis can be obtained in companies, with the objective of raising awareness of the issues. While intended for company executives, this guide is not meant as a stand-alone, but should lead to collective consideration involving line management, occupational physicians and employees' representatives. The presence of trained presenters will improve its efficiency.

4.4. "Age Management. Growing Older while Working", GILLES M., LOISIL Fl., éditions de l'ANACT, 2003

Age management concerns not only seniors, but also all other age groups in the company. Even at a young age one can yet be too old for certain activities where workload or time management are too restricting. The aim of this work is to use real case studies to show how companies can make work more widely accessible, whatever the age, without any loss in performance, avoiding work-related physical problems and exhaustion or exclusion. It presents action road maps to redesign working situations, bringing together organisation, work, time organisation, training, and career management.

Germany

Reinhold Sochert

<table>
<tr><th>Field of promotion</th><th>Physical strain</th><th>Psyche / cognition</th><th>Mental / social competence</th><th>Professional competence</th></tr>
<tr><td>Action</td><td colspan="4"></td></tr>
<tr><td>Relief of physical strain / WHP actions</td><td colspan="2">Setting-based measures</td><td></td><td></td></tr>
<tr><td></td><td colspan="2">Behaviour-based measures *</td><td></td><td></td></tr>
<tr><td></td><td colspan="3">Age-specific risk assessment</td><td></td></tr>
<tr><td></td><td colspan="4">Adapted work-design and working conditions to suit ageing worker's performance</td></tr>
<tr><td></td><td colspan="3">In-house nursery school</td><td></td></tr>
<tr><td></td><td colspan="4">Implementing age management solution as part of HR policy</td></tr>
<tr><td></td><td colspan="4">Teams of mixed age or know-how teams</td></tr>
<tr><td></td><td colspan="4">Better age composition / balance of workforce</td></tr>
<tr><td></td><td colspan="4">HR concepts for more than one generation</td></tr>
<tr><td></td><td colspan="4">Changes in vocational task in order to promote health</td></tr>
<tr><td>Age-related working hours</td><td colspan="3">Reduction of working hours for older workers</td><td></td></tr>
<tr><td></td><td colspan="3">Better reconciliation of family and job within diversity management: part-time work</td><td></td></tr>
<tr><td></td><td colspan="3">Better reconciliation of family and job within diversity management: telecommuting</td><td></td></tr>
<tr><td></td><td colspan="3">Systematic over-all limit on shift working in one's professional life</td><td></td></tr>
<tr><td>Qualification</td><td colspan="4">Support for further training for employees from the age of 50 on</td></tr>
</table>

<table>
<tr><th>Field of promotion</th><th>Physical strain</th><th>Psyche / cognition</th><th>Mental / social competence</th><th>Professional competence</th></tr>
<tr><td></td><td></td><td colspan="3">Adapted training environments to promote special learning skills of aged workers</td></tr>
<tr><td></td><td colspan="4">Better and more guided exchange of knowledge and experience between generations</td></tr>
<tr><td></td><td></td><td colspan="3">Flexible training system to qualify and integrate older unemployed</td></tr>
<tr><td></td><td colspan="4">Altering the youth-centred towards an experienced-centred innovation strategy</td></tr>
<tr><td></td><td colspan="4">New organisation and staff development concepts for longer productive employment</td></tr>
<tr><td>Communication</td><td colspan="4">Quick check "Working longer more healthy"</td></tr>
<tr><td></td><td colspan="4">"Guideline for self-analysing of age structure problems in companies"</td></tr>
<tr><td></td><td colspan="4">Identifying fields of action: start of career, staff development, health, end of career</td></tr>
<tr><td></td><td colspan="4">Better communication between departments and the like</td></tr>
<tr><td></td><td colspan="4">Sensitisation of management and workforce for the cause
(incl. worker's council, works meeting, employers)</td></tr>
<tr><td></td><td colspan="4">Communicating messages on older employees:
special strengths, appropriate work-design, learning, promoting health</td></tr>
<tr><td></td><td colspan="4">Media campaign (posters, press service, ads, events)
for modern OSH - on the key issue "Working longer more healthy"</td></tr>
</table>

** Exercise, nutrition, consumption of alcohol and nicotine, relaxation*

Fig. 8: Summary of actions - Germany

1. Political basis

1.1. Labour Market Policy

Companies can exploit numerous subsidy possibilities in Germany when they decide on further training for older workers, use part-time and retirement/part-time models for older employees, and/or recruit older unemployed people in their company. To this end there is a wide range of tools available to the companies according to the Social Security Code III (SGB III), the Act on Part-time Work for Those Approaching Pensionable Age (AtG) and the Part-Time and Limited Contract Act (TzBfG). The first and second laws for modern services on the labour market ("Hartz I" and "Hartz II") dated January 1, 2003, have resulted in further innovations, especially for older employees:

- Integration subsidies for older unemployed people (at least six months) from the age of 50 (SGB III).
- Support for the further training of employees over 50 years in companies with generally less than 100 workers (SGB III).
- Exemption of the employer from paying contributions to the unemployment insurance fund when an unemployed person over 55 years is recruited (SGB III).
- Integration subsidies, grants for work aids and cost reimbursements for older employees with disabilities from the age of 50 (SGB III).
- Improved possibility to limit the employment contracts of older employees aged 52 and over (TzBfG).
- Tax exemptions, social security privileges and grants from the Labour Exchange for part-time/pensionable workers from the age of 55 (AtG).
- Safeguarding remuneration of older unemployed people from the age of 50 (SGB III).
- Cutting the time for receiving unemployment benefit from max. 32 months to 18 months from the age of 55 (law on "reforms on the labour market", 2003).

- Employer's obligation to pay back the unemployment benefit for up to two years on dismissing a long-standing employee from the age of 55 (law on "reforms on the labour market", 2003).

2. National programmes / projects

2.1. Initiative New Quality of Work (INQA)

The Initiative New Quality of Work (INQA) is an alliance involving the federal government, state governments, social insurance funds, and management and labour foundations. With INQA (www.inqa.de) the initiative partners want to link the interest of people in positive, health- and personality-enhancing working conditions with the need for competitive jobs. INQA is divided up into different initiative issue groups (Thematische Initiativkreise - TIKs); of special interest is the TIK "Ageing in Employment".

The initiative group Ageing in Employment is a platform for disseminating knowledge, experience and activities to improve the work ability of older employees and for different contributions to this topic. The aim of this TIK is to provide appreciable assistance towards conditions furthering the employment of ageing workers.

Key issues are:

- Information about older employees (geared to the target group) concerning how to work out and communicate their special strengths, address challenges in the design of work, special aspects for learning and special activities for maintaining and promoting health at work.
- Collating examples of good practice and ensuring they are disseminated.
- Publicising, using and evaluating tools and activities which can be deployed in company practice in order to boost the employability of older workers.
- Creation of a network of proactive people and bodies to safeguard the objectives of the TIK in the long term.

In 2004, the campaign 30,40,50plus was launched, mainly geared to the first key issue (communication of information on older employees). For this purpose two brochures and a memorandum were prepared. The campaign is being continued in 2005.

2.2. Transfer Project "PR and Marketing Strategy of Demographic Change (Demotrans)"

The aim of the project, sponsored by the Federal Ministry for Education and Research from 1999 to May 2002, was to publicise research results on the demographic change and the world of work by means of this transfer project and to actively market the results within the target groups. The project had recourse to a host of results from long-standing activities sponsored by the Federal Ministry for Education and Research. These were made available to enterprises, associations, politicians and the public as a guide for their activities. In addition, 14 sub-projects on important issues of demographic change were funded, aiming at the development of practicable solutions.

The key issues are:

- safeguarding the ability to work and be innovative,
- HR policy for all age groups,
- health + competence = performance, and
- demanding employability - promoting employment.

In order to achieve the goal of maintaining the health of older employees, an action guide on participation-oriented health management was prepared. Other products are organisation and staff development concepts for longer productive employment in enterprises. These also contain concepts for changes in tasks in order to promote health.

During the course of the project, various networks and follow-up projects were set up which were concerned with individual project results so that the issue was continuously dealt with. Although the project itself has been completed, the website still exists and thus continues to pursue the objective of transferring the results to enterprises and the general public. (www.demotrans.de/)

2.3. EQUAL - Campaign for Older Persons

Innovative approaches to combat discrimination and inequality on the labour market are being tested in Europe within the community initiative EQUAL, financed by € 3 billion of European social fund money. As one of over a hundred development partnerships in Germany, the Campaign for Older Persons (www.offensive-fuer-aeltere.de/) - a group of 17 partners from the welfare sector, research, and business - is compiling strategies against the exclusion of older persons from the labour market. The Campaign for Older Persons aims to reconstitute employability, create new jobs and develop a flexible training system. The campaign also joins a lively exchange of work experience and results together with common activities in a transnational partnership with France, Italy and Sweden. The German partner of the campaign is the Regional Association of Free Welfare Maintenance (LAG) in North Rhine-Westphalia (NRW). Action 1, the planning period, ended in May 2002, subsequently followed by action 2, in which the partners will hold concrete training courses to qualify and integrate older unemployed people. These measures have an integrated approach and will explicitly include the employers. The campaign for older persons will act as an open group for its duration and will complete its work with action 3, when their results will be disseminated in the labour market policy at a federal and community level with the help of "alliance for labour". The development partnership is scientifically monitored and evaluated.

2.4. Gemeinschaftsinitiative Gesünder Arbeiten e. V. (GiGA)

In February 2001, companies (both staff and management), Berufsgenossenschaften (institutions for statutory accident insurance and prevention) and health insurance funds joined forces with the Ministry of Economics and Labour to increasingly highlight a modern understanding of occupational safety and health in the public eye and to implement it in companies. The starting point was a feasibility study which was sponsored by the European Union and the state of North Rhine-Westphalia. It showed that one promising strategy is to draw the attention of companies and workers - by using theme work and PR methods - to modern, preventive, holistic, health-oriented occupational safety and health which is successfully integrated into the company procedures. On this basis, Gemeinschaftsinitiative (GiGA - www.gesuenderarbeiten.de/) advertises publicly with posters, press services, advertisements, events and other media for modern occupational safety and health: information folders and brochures provide information on key issues such as "mobbing", "stress", "user-friendly software" or "Working longer more healthily". One of GiGA's current projects is a quick check on the subject of "Working longer more healthily". This check - aimed at a future-oriented HR policy - is to support companies in estimating the prospective viability of their HR policy. The "Best Practice Award" presented by GiGA rewards exemplary occupational safety and health projects pursued in small and medium-sized enterprises in NRW. Among those rewarded are also five company examples which originate from the national "Demographic Initiative" sponsored by the Federal Ministry of Education and Research (BMBF - see also 4.2.1.-4.2.5.).

2.5. arbid - Work and Innovation in Demographic Change

Being aware that company competitiveness and maintaining jobs is a general concern, the social partners have joined the Ministry for Industry and Labour in North Rhine Westphalia to work out an initiative on work and innovation in demographic change called "arbid". They assume that both employers and employees have common interests in coming to terms with the demographic changes and expect that necessary restructuring can be accomplished more easily by cooperation between the employers' associations and the unions. arbid wants to help as many companies as possible to recognise the advantages as well as the risks involved in the demographic change. Competent contact partners should be made available for companies in the associations, unions, and at educational and advisory centres in NRW. Models of good practice, successful strategies and reliable methods should be further disseminated. (http://www.arbid.de/)

3. Players

3.1. NGOs / interest group representatives

3.1.1. PROage - Facing the Challenge of Demographic Change

The Confederation of the German Employers' Associations initiated the project "PROage" (www.proage-online.de/) in autumn 2001, together with the Bertelsmann Foundation as well as three European employers' associations from Denmark, the Netherlands and Ireland with the support of the European Commission. The aim of the project was to develop - in a dialogue with representatives from politics, science and industry - action-oriented approaches and strategies to tackle the imminent demographic shortage of workforce and to draw public awareness more to the need for longer personal employment biographies. In addition to transnational expert seminars, two scientific studies were commissioned. An international comparison of the statutory and collectively agreed conditions for the employment of older workers - "More employment opportunities for older workers - International comparison and recommendations" - and also a compendium of models of good practice - "Successful with older employees - Strategies and examples for in-company practice" - were published. At the final international conference in Berlin on September 25, 2003, the project's concepts for raising older workers' participation in employment were publicly presented and possibilities for their implementation in politics and company practice explained.

3.1.2. Industry-Wide Metalworkers' Union (IG-Metall)

The focal points of the work of IG-Metall to improve the employment of older workers are:

- age-specific risk assessment,
- pursuing model projects for the design of work to suit ageing workers and promote their learning skills,
- anchoring of qualification planning and further training in the enterprises, and
- HR planning to suit an ageing workforce.

To this end specialised events, workshops, company projects, cooperation and work aids are planned. (www.igmetall.de/)

3.1.3. Combined Services Trade Union (VERDI)

For the trade union VERDI, the approach to solving the demographic problems is to be found in a different economic policy. For example, according to VERDI, the effects of demographic shifts could be offset by an extension of gainful employment and a different distribution of the production profits. In order to raise the employment rate of older workers, working conditions would have to be changed so that work can still be performed by older people.

A systematic time limit on shift work during one's work biography would be conceivable for VERDI. Moreover, VERDI stresses the significance of the demographic change for workplace health promotion as well as for labour and HR policies to suit older workers.

A survey was conducted aimed at people who had left employment. It dealt with the future possibilities of a healthy transition into retirement. Results of the survey will be publicised in 2005. (www.verdi.de/)

3.1.4. Central Association of the Sanitary Heating and Air Conditioning Industry (ZVSHK)

The focal points of a project related to ageing workers were potential company solutions. They were also listed as examples of good practice:

- offers of further training,
- improvement in work and company organisation.
- promotion of management and HR management, and
- recruitment of qualified staff.

The following conclusion can be drawn: the intensive collaboration laid a foundation for further labour- and HR-policies in companies to suit an ageing workforce. Continuity and sustainability are guaranteed by the know-how transfer between the ZVSHK, the SHK organisations and the trade and skilled crafts as a whole (ZdH - German Confederation of Skilled Crafts). The further implementation of proposed solutions is driven by the advisory and design activities of the IAP - Institute for work design and personnel management (e.g. qualification concepts for older employees in trade and crafts) and of the ZVSHK (e.g. training concept "HR concepts for more than one generation"). The ZVSHK and its partners supported 47 companies in the implementation of concepts for company activities and strategies to tackle the demographic change. (www.wasserwaermeluft.de/)

3.1.5. Central Association of the Electrical Engineering and Electronics Industries (ZVEI)

The consulting concept of the ZVEI/GfAH is designed as a "guideline for the self-analysis of age structure problems in companies". In 12 chapters, information is given on how the "workforce of the future", the "age structures" and a "broad range of HR solutions" can be determined and developed:

1) The age gap
2) Early warning indicators
3) Age structure analysis
4) Balanced age HR policy
5) Recruitment strategies
6) Company loyalty
7) Early retirement
8) Learning for life
9) Career development
10) Knowledge transfer
11) Health care
12) Respect culture

Conclusion of the project: To tackle the future problems, target oriented changes which can take place step by step over prolonged periods are important. This restructuring of HR policy can be performed in several ways, by means of a reorientation towards positive examples, generating future scenarios or the processing of targeted tasks to determine the future HR strategy. 30 companies were involved in this project. (www.zvei.org/demografie/)

3.1.6. German Machinery and Plant Manufacturers Association (VDMA)

The advisory concept of the VDMA comprises two stages:

- Sensitisation of management and workforce for the subject "Ageing at Work".

In order to sensitise the management in large companies, aspects such as "economic efficiency", "costs and earnings" are highlighted; for the management in small and medium-sized enterprises ("a matter for the boss") references are made to "age structure analyses" and "threat scenarios". The workforce has to be involved by the inclusion of the workers' council, works meetings and dialogues with the employees.

- Possible company solutions in four fields of action.

On the basis of talks and consultancy with the companies the most urgent problem areas and thus fields of action were determined in the enterprises. For these four fields of action (start of career, staff development, health, end of career) specific materials and possible solutions were offered on which the enterprises could then hammer out their own activities. An integrated action strategy is available to enterprises which want to act in all four fields.

Conclusion: In some companies the subject of demography was the vehicle to start or put forward the process of modernisation (reorganisation, restructuring of corporate culture). By dealing with the change in age structure, quite a few companies started to illustrate their workforce structure systematically according to certain criteria and, based on this, their staff development. Roughly 40 enterprises participated in the project. (www.vdma.de/)

3.2. Private / commercial service enterprises

3.2.1. ARÖW - Association for Work, Reorganisation and Ecological Economic Counselling GmbH

ARÖW links innovation research and counselling in specific branches and areas of work. 20 members of staff also advise enterprises on how to introduce company age management. The initiative AGE-Management aims at sensitising companies and administrations for problems which the German economy is likely to face in the near future and to prepare managements for new tasks. Experts from various disciplines joined forces for this project. These experts offer supportive services for organisations in industry, trade/skilled crafts and administration: when consulted, the company's individual situation is analysed and tailor-made AGE-Management solutions are worked out. Establishment of regional experts' networks of the initiative AGE-Management is backed by funds from the state of NRW and the European Union. (www.aroew.de/)

3.2.2. prospektiv - Gesellschaft für Betriebliche Zukunftsgestaltungen mbH

prospektiv GmbH, a research and consulting company based in Dortmund since 1996, currently employs 14 staff members. Their range comprises consulting services on issues of staff and organisation development, occupational safety and health and strategic corporate development. In order to offer scientifically proven concepts, research projects are also initiated and implemented.

In the business fields "Staff and Organisation Development" and "Occupational Safety and Health" the company focuses on issues and services related to HR activities for handling ageing workforces. Performance of age structure analyses and strategic HR management (prevention, work organisation, career development) is monitored. (www.prospektiv.de/)

3.3. Research organisations

3.3.1. Gesellschaft für Arbeitsschutz- und Humanisierungsforschung mbH Volkholz und Partner (GfAH)

GfAH is a privately run institute concentrating on research and consultancy in work and social sciences. Approaches to an age-balanced HR policy are of interest. GfAH sees this policy as a re-orientation in HR management towards a better age mixture or age balance in the workforce. The concept of the age-balanced HR policy allows for the different interests and needs of younger and older workers. One element in the institute's concept is a tool for age structure analysis which GfAH has developed. (www.gfah.de/)

3.3.2. Forschungsgesellschaft für Gerontologie e.V.

This research company for gerontology was set up in Dortmund in the early 1990s. The company's aim was to create an initial starting point for research and consulting needs related to social gerontology. In addition to the state of NRW and the City of Dortmund, over 50 renowned institutions and reputable individuals from politics, science and practice are members of the Forschungsgesellschaft für Gerontologie. Forschungsgesellschaft für Gerontologie has been running the Institute for Gerontology for the conception and implementation of socio-gerontological research projects in practice since 1992. The range comprises research and consulting projects in the following fields:

- demographic change and the world of work,
- health and care research, and
- life situation research and age social policy.

(www.uni-dortmund.de/FFG/)

3.3.3. Sozialforschungsstelle Dortmund (sfs)

Sozialforschungsstelle Dortmund is one of the major German institutes for labour research. Founded back in 1946, sfs has been a federal state institute since 1972. It is assigned to the Ministry for Science and Research of the state of NRW. In addition to application-oriented fundamental research, e.g. on work organisation and occupational safety and health, Sozialforschungsstelle offers advice on new production concepts or on further vocational training and evaluates the introduction of eco-audits. Studies on the consequences of multimedia technologies are conducted. The institute deals with aspects of labour market policy, specific to women and older workers, and with health policy as well as with the future of codetermination. Roughly 50 scientific employees (social scientists, economists, pedagogues, statisticians, engineers and information scientists) work at Sozialforschungsstelle in eight areas of research. The research field "Work and health" focuses on age(ing)-appropriate work in small enterprises. (www.sfs-dortmund.de)

3.3.4. Institut für Sozialforschung und Sozialwirtschaft Saarbrücken (iso)

Established in 1969, the iso institute is an autonomous and independent social scientific research facility employing roughly 15 scientists (social sciences, economics, psychology, political sciences). It has been successfully operating in research and consultancy for 35 years. Clients of the institute are predominantly Federal Ministries (BMBF - Federal Ministry for Education and Research, BMGS - Federal Ministry for Health and Social Security, BMFSFJ - Federal Ministry for Families, Seniors, Women and Youth, BMWA - Federal Ministry for Work and Economy), but also state ministries, foundations, the European Commission, local authorities, associations, chambers and companies in the private sector from industry and the services' sector. The focal point of the iso institute's work is application-oriented, socio-scientific research. In addition, it pursues fundamental research and - based on the results of the application-oriented research - also offers consulting services. iso researches and offers advice on topics like "World of Work and Health" and "The Elderly" for which numerous projects on the issue of "Age and Health" have been and are currently conducted.
(www.iso-institut.de/)

3.3.5. Fraunhofer-Institut für Arbeitswirtschaft und Organisation (IAO)

The activities of the Fraunhofer Institute for Industrial Engineering (IAO) focus on the investigation of current topics in the field of technology management. A holistic approach is applied to the study of commercial success, employees' interests and social consequences. In keeping with the holistic approach, attention is given to the individual and social values held by people in their working environment. This addresses the task of creating ergonomic solutions and also the additional qualifications required by employees in coping with the decentralised organisation of work and the implementation of new technologies. Research projects are conducted in close collaboration with small and medium-sized companies and industrial corporations under direct contract. The Fraunhofer IAO participates in publicly funded research programmes, such as the "Information Technology" and "Work and Technology" programmes of the German Federal Ministry of Education and Research, in programmes of the European Union as well as in programmes funded by the county of Baden-Württemberg.

The transfer and implementation project "Public Relations and Marketing Strategy of Demographic Change" (see 2.2. Demotrans) is an integrated project consisting of 14 sub-projects and is coordinated and marketed by the Fraunhofer IAO. (www.iao.fhg.de/)

4. Projects

4.1. Industry / larger companies

4.1.1. Ford-Werke AG

At Ford-Werke AG diversity is a central element of the corporate strategy and culture. Diversity concentrates on the differences as well as on the common aspects of people and the integration of workers. Diversity management is a successful approach to staff development. At Ford-Werke AG this includes, for example, activities which aim to increase the proportion of women in technical jobs (participation at Girls' Day of the Federal Ministry for Education and Research, cooperation with universities). The reconciliation of family and job is another element in diversity management. For example, part-time work and telework are offered, in addition to Ford's own nursery school. Employees with disabilities are also a separate target group.

For this purpose Ford has its own disability management. The task of the disability manager is to integrate employees with disabilities back into production and give them comprehensive advice on ergonomic measures. The manager ensures the implementation of the aforementioned measures at the workplace and can also propose prevention and health promotion activities. (www.ford.de/)

4.1.2. Stahlwerke Bremen

Stahlwerke Bremen is a steel mill (flat steel products) belonging to the ARBED group with roughly 5,000 employees. In 1995, a model trial was initiated on the re-integration of older employees with an occupational disability into the company workflows. In 1998, the model was assessed and continued by other works since 1999. Employees affected remain in the company during the project but are accompanied by the Society for Health and Rehabilitation of Stahlwerke Bremen.

Measures in the model project are:

- performance potential analysis,
- brief qualifications, and
- working trials.

(www.stahlwerke-bremen.de/)

4.1.3. SCHOTT Jenaer Glas GmbH

The JENA GmbH is a company rich in tradition in the glass industry and was founded in 1884. Since 1990, the company has belonged to the SCHOTT Group whose headquarters are located in Mainz. In the years after German re-unification the company underwent a fundamental upheaval and now employs 650 workers, including 170 women. The result of surveys and discussions as part of a workshop showed the following problem areas with the need for action:

- everyday work and testing new things are too close together ("daily business overwhelms"),
- cooperation and communication in the company are not optimal - in particular concerning the introduction of new products, and
- there is too little systematic and targeted exchange of knowledge and experience between the generations.

Therefore:
- suggestions for an improvement scheme should be further developed,
- the imminent gap in skilled workers and experience should be counteracted, and
- the market and product strategy should be designed to be more aggressive.

In the subsequent project group work with twelve employees from all departments, potential solutions for two problem areas were sought and found:
- an improvement in cooperation and communication between the departments (development, production, sales), and
- a more targeted exchange of knowledge and experience between generations should be aspired.

At the end of 2001 a positive conclusion was first drawn from the results of the project group work and recommendations on the continuation of the change process were passed on to the divisional management. Secondly, with the results achieved, the project group participated in the pan-Group competition for improvement teams. (http://www.schott.com/jena/german/)

4.2. Electrical engineering and electronics industry / small and medium-sized enterprises

4.2.1. ABB Automation Products (APR) GmbH, Minden

The company belongs to ABB AG Deutschland and manufactures products for instrumentation and control technology with a workforce of 500 (in 2002). Studies conducted as part of the company's demography initiative pointed towards the fact that the imminent staff changes (over-ageing, gaps in workforce) could not be overcome by conventional HR strategies (5-year plan with one- to two-year operational plans).

It was shown that in years to come, long term planning horizons were indispensable in order to harmonise initial training, new recruits, part-time work/early retirement schemes, staff development and health programmes in terms of objectives and timing. The HR management therefore worked out and implemented a 10-year plan as a new tool for HR work. This plan will safeguard the know-how transfer from older to younger employees, and also sustain the employability of the current workforce with measures for maintaining health and qualification until they reach retirement age. Furthermore, APR is intensifying its activities to win new skilled workers, not only by means of an improved training concept but also by increasing cooperation with schools and universities. (www.abb.com)

4.2.2. Brähler International Congress Service (ICS) AG, Königswinter

In 2002, Brähler employed 127 workers in Germany. ICS AG is a solution provider for communications media. The medium-sized enterprise operates in over 80 countries. 70 % of its employees are skilled workers, 20 % university graduates and 10 % unskilled or trained workers. Owing to the low labour turnover rate of only 1 %, continuous recruitment and a currently young to middle-aged workforce, the proportion of older workers will increase significantly in the medium term. It has to be expected that roughly two thirds of the workforce will be 50 years or over in ten years' time. Maintaining the employability of these workers is thus becoming a key issue for the company.

Maintaining health and - above all - further qualification of the ageing workforce are the key tasks of the HR management. Personal and company-wide qualification concepts for the existing team will serve as a basis for developing the necessary fields of knowledge in the high-tech area. To be able to implement the training offensive, activities to promote motivation and personal initiative are being started. (www.braehler.com)

4.2.3. Digitale Repro-Systeme (DRS) GmbH, Oberhausen

The company employs 6 workers (2002) and was set up by experts of different disciplines in 1998, to develop, manufacture and market innovative digitisation equipment and the related services worldwide. The core team is middle-aged and older. The oldest workers are over 50. A simple extrapolation for the next 10 years is not readily possible but would result in substantial age structure problems. The start-up company DRS has therefore developed long-term staff planning and uniform staff principles which offer a common basis for action while in consolidation.

Special features are measures to prevent self-exploitation among the motivated staff and to win new skilled workers to supplement them as part of successor planning. Aspects of internal communications and cooperation are promoted in particular as well as the integration of independent workers and freelancers recruited from a network with other small and medium-sized enterprises. (www.drs-online.de)

4.2.4. NanoFocus AG, Oberhausen

NanoFocus specialises in the development, production and marketing of 3D measuring instruments and has 32 employees (in 2002). As a former start-up company, NanoFocus has now reached a size which necessitates consolidation. Cost management, standardisation, reliability, empirical knowledge and an awareness of responsibility are in demand. Moreover, by the year 2012, further projected growth to 102 workers in Germany and 40 in foreign sales companies is planned. In the age structure of 2002, one third of the employees were 45 years old and beyond, two thirds were under 45 years. Given a simple extrapolation up to 2012, a structure centred on middle-aged workers will be produced from this distribution with a "peak" among the 25-34-year-olds. NanoFocus has been geared to a balanced age composition for years. To be able to shape growth and internal consolidation in a balanced manner, the necessary different key qualifications are to be merged in suitable forms of cooperation and communication. A successor arrangement which kicks in at an early stage ensures the familiarisation of younger workers with the work. To improve company loyalty, various bonus models will be introduced in the years to come. Qualification plans serve to maintain the staff level.
(www.nanofocus.de)

4.2.5. microTEC Gesellschaft für Mikrotechnologie mbH, Duisburg/Bad Dürkheim

microTEC operates in the field of batch production of micro-system products without tooling and employs 22 workers (in 2002). With the fast-growing company microTEC, looking after ageing workers must be combined with the recruitment of other employees. Professional and social integration is achieved through benefit partnerships in teams of mixed ages. In doing so, interesting observations on mutual acceptance and self-understanding as well as on the learning behaviour of the individual workers were made. The HR management strategy comprises specific aims for recruitment, an integrative corporate philosophy and steps towards improving the working situation, which have, for the large part, already been implemented.
(www.microtec-d.com)

4.2.6. Advising Software-Developing Companies on the Consequences of the Change in Age Structure

The subject of this project is to prepare concepts, models and possibilities for the design of work situations for software developers aged over 40 years with the aim of promoting this age group and safeguarding their employment possibilities in the long term.

The project relates to a branch of industry - software development - which in recent years has become the epitome of the exclusion of older workers and of youth-centred staff structures. Against the backdrop of a development in which competitiveness is being increasingly determined by experience with projects and the customers, the project is aimed at changing the youth-centred innovation strategy towards an experience-centred innovation strategy.

Proposed activities in the following fields of action were worked out in the project to achieve better inclusion of older software developers:

- career planning,
- roles for older software developers, and
- innovative further training management.

Concepts and action guides, such as check lists and guidelines, were developed in each of these fields of action.
(http://www.physik.tu-cottbus.de/ztg/Techphil/)

4.3. Public administration / services

4.3.1. Munich Municipal Services - Division Transport Operations

A driver's job is a high-stress profession with a high risk of illness and high sickness rates; it is not very attractive and therefore has problems with young recruits. Many of the drivers are taken out of service at the age of 49 owing to their acquired unsuitability for driving. They are then transferred to office work, which is both unpopular and uneconomic. The aim of the programme of the Munich transport operations division was to help reduce the unsuitability for driving service, cut lost days, prolong the time drivers remained in driving service, increase attraction and improve customer orientation. The PE-GF (staff development/health promotion) programme was started in

1993, at that time still run by the local authority, on the initiative of staff representatives and the occupational physician. The City of Munich had already declared its willingness to bear the high staff replacement costs. The programme has been the largest in Germany and is still continued today by the HR management in a privatised company (plc). The programme had three effective levers:

- training,
- group process, and
- reduction in working time.

(http://www.mvv-muenchen.de)

4.3.2. Deutsche Bank AG

Age diversity is one of Deutsche Bank's main global diversity initiative issues. It is based on the vision of demonstrating industry leadership by fostering an inclusive work environment in which all employees contribute to their full potential and diverse teams maximise their performance. The bank considers this as essential for a true meritocracy, increased shareholder value and greater profitability. Management of age diversity means that the bank's business and HR strategy is focused on all age groups and takes into consideration their individual demands for personal development, career, working practice and job design. Cooperation between different age groups is a necessary and important prerequisite for the success of teams, while managers are responsible for creating an inclusive work environment for all age groups. Age-related initiatives at Deutsche Bank focus primarily on the aspects

- employability,
- training,
- mentoring, and
- advanced professionals programmes.

There are several working models in the bank to support experienced employees in learning and the sharing of experiences between different generations, e.g. intergenerational project teams or know-how teams. This model was used to develop customer contact and acquisition skills, facilitate transfer of IT-related knowledge, and optimise the process of customer handover. (www.deutsche-bank.de/)

4.4. Networks

4.4.1. GENERA - The Young and the Old: Workforce Integration as an Organisational Task

As part of the EQUAL project (see also 2.3. EQUAL - Campaign for Older Persons), players from the foundry and forging industry - above all the German Foundry Association and the trade union IG Metall - joined forces in the development partnership GENERA to solve urgent problems of HR management in these two industrial branches: the excessive ageing of the workforces (an average age of 50 is not uncommon) and the major problems in winning young recruits at all levels. Together with the currently 17 pilot-, consulting- and qualification-companies, the network project is working on the following tasks:

- Maintaining and increasing the efficiency of older workers, who are frequently semiskilled or unskilled, through new forms of furthered vocational training and by work organisation appropriate for older workers.
- Opening up the branches to groups which had previously not been in the focus of their activities. Here, migrants from Eastern Europe, women (previously heavily underrepresented) and people with "broken" work biographies were aimed at. They are specially prepared for work in specific companies of the branch.
- This is connected with activities aimed at improving the image of the branch and in particular at further increasing the presence in the regions and on regional labour markets.

The development partnership GENERA has a sectoral approach with focus on NRW. However, companies from other German provinces (Thuringia, Saxony, Baden-Württemberg, Rhineland-Palatinate, Lower Saxony, Hesse) are also participating. Overall coordination is done with Soziale Innovation GmbH, a consulting and research facility in Dortmund. The German Foundry Association coordinates all the activities at branch level. (www.genera-info.de)

4.4.2. Network for Age-Appropriate Work - NETAB

This network project has also been pursued under the joint initiative EQUAL (see also 2.3. EQUAL - Campaign for Older Persons). Under the management of the Educational Network of Lower Saxony Adult Education Centres (BNVHS), partners from industry, science, further education institutions, chambers, and public organisations have joined to form the "Network for Age-Appropriate Work - NETAB". The eight operational partners (incl. Volkswagen AG) are responsible for implementing the agenda. They receive advice and support from ten strategic partners (incl. IG Metall), which provide important momentum in regions or sectors and have already built a network for the dissemination of information and values.

The aim of the network is to achieve a turnabout in HR policy for handling ageing workforces. In particular, NETAB is working on the following issues and projects:

- developing practical answers and examples worth emulating,
- demonstrating new approaches, e.g. through a concept of company self-analysis,
- combating prejudice towards older workers and calling people to assume responsibility, and
- contributing towards counteracting the demographic and industrial changes through information, advice, qualification and project support.

(www.netab.de)

Hungary

Ferenc Kudász

<table>
<tr><th>Field of promotion</th><th>Physical strain</th><th>Psyche / cognition</th><th>Mental / social competence</th><th>Professional competence</th></tr>
<tr><td>Action</td><td colspan="4"></td></tr>
<tr><td>Relief of physical strain / WHP actions</td><td colspan="3">Fitness-for-job examinations</td><td></td></tr>
<tr><td></td><td colspan="3">Behaviour-based actions * - "Healthy lifestyle" package</td><td></td></tr>
<tr><td></td><td colspan="3">Reduction of hard physical work, especially under hazardous conditions</td><td></td></tr>
<tr><td></td><td colspan="3">Avoidance of unapt ergonomic situations</td><td></td></tr>
<tr><td></td><td></td><td colspan="2">Mental health promotion incl.:</td><td></td></tr>
<tr><td></td><td colspan="4">Time management</td></tr>
<tr><td></td><td colspan="3">Conflict management</td><td></td></tr>
<tr><td></td><td colspan="4">Stress prevention</td></tr>
<tr><td>Age-related working hours</td><td colspan="3">Increasing the rate of holidays from 20 to 30 days by the age of 45</td><td></td></tr>
<tr><td>Qualification</td><td></td><td></td><td></td><td></td></tr>
<tr><td>Communication</td><td colspan="4">Activities for fellowship reinforcement</td></tr>
<tr><td></td><td colspan="4">Publishing a guide for models of good practice</td></tr>
<tr><td></td><td colspan="4">Better cooperation of experts organising WHP activities</td></tr>
<tr><td></td><td colspan="4">Lobbying for the case of WHP by the hungarian federation of mutual funds</td></tr>
<tr><td></td><td colspan="4">Installing elements of WHP in collective agreements</td></tr>
</table>

** Exercise, nutrition, consumption of alcohol and nicotine, relaxation*

Fig. 9: Summary of actions - Hungary

1. National programmes / projects

1.1. The Public Health Programme for the Healthy Nation (2001-2010)

Hungarian legislation has recently approved the "National Programme of Work Safety" (MOP) for the institutional development of work safety and the "Public Health Programme for the Healthy Nation" to improve the population's health. These programmes stress the different priorities in work protection and public health policies.

Not only influencing life style, but developing "supportive workplace environment" and health promotion as well, is among the strategic goals in long term projects in the Public Health Programme. Up to the year 2010, a sub-programme for establishing a healthier environment defines objectives to research and prevent the harmful effects caused by work and the working environment. Fundamental to this programme are the data collected about population, work hygiene and occupational health services. This will enable the establishment and development of exposure- and morbidity-registers, databases for National Health Care Services, chemical safety databases and informational systems. As the programme has only been established recently, no data or databases are available so far.

Following the governmental change in 2002, the programme was left in abeyance, but in 2003, the new Government monitored and modified the programme by setting new aims and objectives. It was named after Johan Béla who achieved outstanding results in Hungarian public health between WWI and WWII.

1.2. National Programme of the Decade of Health "Johan Béla"

The parliamentary decree No. 46/2003 gives the aim of the programme as the improvement of the currently very poor state of health of the Hungarian population (e.g. life expectancy at birth: 76 years for females, 68 for males). Thus it has the subtitle "health promotion in everyday life". Parliament demands that Hungarian workplaces should emphasise health promotion even beyond the mandatory work health measures.

In 2003, 15 competitors were awarded financial support and the title "Healthy Workplace" in the field of workplace health promotion. In 2004, 18 competitors won this title. To do this, they had to assemble and tender a dossier of the realisation of definite WHP programmes. The view-points of the jury were based mainly on the ENWHP criteria.

The main aim of this activity is the creation of a guide for models of good practice. The first invitation to compete for the award was announced in the official state health bulletin - "Egészségügyi Közlöny" - thus the applicants were mainly health and social care institutions such as schools and hospitals. In the future, the involvement of local governments and ministries is expected.

1.3. The Nationwide Programme of Work Safety (MOP - A Munkavédelem Országos Programja)

The decree No. 20/2001 on MOP lays down fundamental long-term strategic principles of workplace health improvement, principles of sustainable development, precaution, prevention and the principle of comprehensive partnership. Each of these principles stresses the importance of health protection and life improvement of workforce, establishing good working atmosphere and health promotion and strengthening social dimensions. These principles are emphasised in a parliamentary act and are in line with multi-sectoral work safety. MOP has set as long-term tasks - amongst others - the objective that efficient work protection systems should be provided customised for individual enterprises and independent accident insurance should be established and serve as a base for workplace health promotion.

Actually the Hungarian health and accident insurance is not a bonus-malus system. Due to scarce capacity of labour safety supervision, workplace checks are rare. This results in labour safety regulations not being thoroughly kept at all. They would be more effective if more rigorously kept.

1.4. The Nationwide Strategy for WHP (*A Munkahelyi Egészségfejlesztés Országos Stratégiája*)

In September 2004, deriving from the latter two programmes, and after completion of a regional analysis, the "Nationwide Strategy" was developed under the guidance of the "National Centre for Health Promotion" and the "Association for Healthier Workplaces". On November 8, 2004, the founding of the "Hungarian Forum for WHP" was accomplished.

1.5. EQUAL Project

On May 28, 2004, the EU project EQUAL, under the guidance of the Ministry of Employment and Labour, was announced - with a deadline in September. Results were expected for December. Among others, the ageing workforce is targeted. Details of the winning projects are to be found at https://equal.cec.eu.int/equal/jsp/index.jsp?lang=de#round. Contracting is taking place at the beginning of 2005.

2. Players

In Hungary, every relevant decision concerning labour issues has to be passed by a tripartite conciliatory council comprising the government and both social partners. Members are delegated from the Ministry of Economy, the Ministry of Finance, certain institutions of work safety, health, social and family matters services. Employees are represented by the significant trade unions (800,000 - 1.200,000 organised workers, 38 %) and finally employers comprising the National Alliance of Employers and Manufacturers (*MGYOSZ*), National Alliance of Entrepreneurs, National Alliance of Strategic Enterprises, Hungarian Alliance of Industry (*OKISZ*), National Alliance of Industrial Chambers (*IPOSZ*), National Alliance of General Consumer Cooperatives (*ÁFEOSZ*), National Interest Protecting Alliance of Retailers and Carriers (*KISOSZ*).

2.1. Governmental organisations

2.1.1. Ministry of Health (Egészségügyi Minisztérium)

The Ministry of Health is the governing institution for the "National Programme of the Decade of Health - Johan Béla" (see 2.2).

2.1.2 Ministry of Employment and Labour (*Foglalkozáspolitikai és Munkaügyi Minisztérium*)

This ministry is co-officer of the "Nationwide Programme of Work Safety" and the "EQUAL" project.

2.1.3. National Centre for Health Promotion (*Országos Egészségfejlesztési Intézet OEFI*)

Founded in 2001, the centre is appointed to be the head-office of national health promotion. Duties include professional, methodological, scientific research- and training-activities. Health Promotion is directed towards the Hungarian population. Support and harmonisation for the programmes of different institutions (NGO and governmental) in the field of health promotion and public health complete the activities.

2.1.4. "Fodor József" Centre for Public Health (*Fodor József Országos Közegészségügyi Központ*)

Founded in 1998, the centre connected institutions to help the Bureau of the Chief Medical Officer (*Országos Tisztiorvosi Hivatal*) on a nationwide basis. It includes the Hungarian NCO for ENWHP (National Institute for Occupational Health - *Országos Munkahigiénés és Foglalkozásegészségügyi Intézet OMFI*), National Institute for Epidemiology (*Országos Epidemiológiai Központ OEK*), National Institute for Environmental Health (*Országos Környezetegészségügyi Intézet OKI*), National Institute for Nutrition and Dietetics (*Országos Élelmezés- és Táplálkozástudományi Intézet OÉTI*), and National Institute for Chemical Safety (*Országos Kémiai Biztonsági Intézet OKBI*).

2.2. Non-governmental Organisations

2.2.1. Association for Healthier Workplaces (*Egészségesebb Munkahelyekért Egyesület*)

In this public benefit organisation, founded in 1997, 25 volunteers encourage workplace health promotion. The association aims at popularising WHP and helps with the use of MOGP. It is a member in the advisory council for WHP in the ministry, founder member of the Hungarian Forum for WHP (*Munkahelyi Egészségfejlesztés Magyarországi Fóruma*) and cooperates with the National Centre for Health Promotion. The chairman of the association took part in the evaluation of the tender for "Healthy Workplace" at the Ministry of Welfare.

The board of the "Association for Healthier Workplace" delegates its members and executives to ENWHP conferences. The Hungarian NCO and the nominated national coordinator are members of the association and its board. Thus they accept the philosophy of ENWHP and also know the proceedings. They recommend not only the Hungarian but also international MsOGP - especially at their meetings, which have become more regular over the last two years.

2.2.2. Hungarian Forum for WHP (*Munkahelyi Egészségfejlesztés Magyarországi Fóruma*)

This task force includes delegates of the National Institute for Occupational Health, National Centre for Health Promotion, Ministry of Health, Association for Healthier Workplaces, Hungarian Federation of Mutual Funds, Occupational Health and Safety Section of the Hungarian Medical Chamber, and the Hungarian Chamber of Engineers. The statutory meeting was held on February 17, 2004, with over 200 participants. 19 enterprises were awarded the title "Health-friendly Workplace" within the scope of the conference. On November 9, the second assembly outlined the "Nationwide Strategy for WHP".

As general targets were given:

1) the activity and cooperation of professionals and value-mediator organisations in the area of WHP should improve,
2) the behaviour, knowledge and activity of workplace performers concerning WHP should progress as widely as possible,
3) the great state systems related to WHP should be harmonised, and
4) the environment of regulations and incentives (legal and financial) should expand.

To accomplish target 1) - among other suggestions - it is proposed to improve skills and utilisation on issues of WHP as well as to develop communication between experts. Additionally, information on the matters of WHP, its access, methods and experiences should gain more publicity.

Concerning target 2) e.g. the concept of health at workplaces should become more standardised and workplace health fund activities should progress.

Target 3) could be achieved by e.g. installing WHP as part of the syllabus of social dialogue and national conciliation. Cooperation could then encourage the development of the tie between preventive and curative care systems and the transfer of emphasis to prevention, whereas the authorities and local governments concerned should augment its role regarding WHP.

Relating to target 4) - amongst others - cooperation is suggested in establishing and harmonising the independent accident insurance system with WHP activities. Hence decision-makers should know WHP related claims and needs of employers and employees. Furthermore suggestions are given for the governmental plan for national development - "Európa Terv" - to incorporate the WHP syllabus in its regional and local development plans. In case of financial benefits, investments in WHP should be widespread, whereas it is proposed to terminate the financial dependence of occupational health services on employers. Prevention and rehabilitation should be augmented in the practical activities of occupational health services and should get more opportunities for implementation in everyday working life.

2.2.3. Hungarian Federation of Mutual Funds (*Magyar Pénztárszövetség*)

The Federation consists of about 60 member organisations, and represents 400,000 individuals. It incorporates a Health Funds Section too. The federation is lobbying for the higher appreciation of health promotion for which fund capital is to be used. They intend to install WHP elements in collective agreements. Both the management and the insured are targeted.

2.2.4. Occupational Health and Safety Section of the Hungarian Medical Chamber (*Magyar Orvosi Kamara, Foglalkozás-egészségügyi Szekció*)

In Hungary, chamber membership is mandatory to medical activity. Occupational health physicians are forming a section within the chamber. Occupational health care is obligatory for organised working activities so the doctors are in attendance in every company. Their skills make them able to participate in WHP. The section in the chamber helps to convince their members of the advantageous effects of WHP and thus the unique society for OHS practitioners acts as partner in the struggle for healthier workplaces.

2.2.5. "Fact" Applied Social Science Research Institution (Fact Intézet)

The privately owned research centre for social research is also involved in work-health studies.

2.2.6. Hungarian Chamber of Engineers (*Magyar Mérnöki Kamara*)

With 400 experts, the Division of Labour Safety (Munkabiztonsági Tagozat) offers opinions on laws and is lobbying for labour safety experts. It cooperates with the OHS Section of the Medical Chamber.

2.2.7. The American Chamber of Commerce in Hungary

The American Chamber of Commerce in Hungary was established in 1989 by 32 American companies as the very first AmCham in Eastern Europe and currently has over 600 members in 22 countries. Their Healthy Workplace Programme was launched in November 2002, and facilitated the spread of Hungarian WHP by implementing good international experiences.

AmCham also established the "Healthy Workplace AmCham Award" by January 2003. This award is offered for AmCham members every year in three categories: corporations, medium-sized companies, small businesses.

There are 14 recommendations, of which some are compulsory, but also optional recommendations need to be fulfilled. Headlines are:

- Development of a healthy working environment: the common handling of health, environment and safety regarding health promotion has to be proved/provided.
- "Live healthily!": this "lifestyle package" comprises the topics:
  - smoking (help in smoke cessation),
  - nutrition (council, information, provision and advocating healthy workplaces), and
  - physical activity (provision of fitness/sport facilities at the workplaces as well as off work).
- Mental health: time management training, conflict handling, stress prevention, activities for fellowship reinforcement.

- Screening program: currently the Hungarian public health system focuses at cardiovascular, metabolic and malignant diseases, but the screening could be extended at musculoskeletal diseases, visual system, weight management etc.

On fulfilling the requirements, the members can display the "Healthy Workplace Certificate" founded and granted by AmCham.

2.3. Training institutions

2.3.1. Semmelweis University (*Semmelweis Egyetem*)

It was integrated from different universities (University of Medicine, University of Physical Training and high schools (High School of Health) to promote a flexible multi-level curriculum. The Department of Work and Environmental Health (*Munka és Környezetegészségügyi Tanszék*) and Institutes of Public Health (university degree *Közegészségügyi Intézet* and high school degree *Népegészségügyi Intézet*) are the main contributors of training for specialists that can meet WHP demands. A one year health promotion course for employees was established at the Institute of Behavioural Medicine (*Magatartástudomány Intézet*). A stress managing "Lifecase" programme of twelve hours is under adaptation for Hungarian conditions. There is also a Ph.D. study on workplace stress and health promotion under way.

2.3.2. University of Pécs (*Pécsi Tudományegyetem*)

The Department of Public Health at the Faculty of Medicine runs an occupational medicine section.

2.3.3. University of Debrecen (*Debreceni Tudományegyetem*)

The School of Public Health at the University of Debrecen runs an M.Sc. course on Health Promotion.

2.3.4. University of Szeged (*Szegedi Tudományegyetem*)

At the Faculty of Teacher Training "Juhász Gyula" the Department of Applied Health Science (*Juhász Gyula Tanárképző Föiskola, Alkalmazott Egészségtudományi Tanszék*) was launched in 1995. Focusing on sociology and psychology, they advocate health promotion training in the field of mental hygiene.

Iceland

Ása Guðbjörg Ásgeirsdóttir

Field of promotion	Physical strain	Psyche / cognition	Mental / social competence	Professional competence
Action				
Relief of physical strain / WHP actions	Setting-based measures			
	Behaviour-based measures *			
Age-related working hours	Decreasing working houres at retirement age			
Qualification	Improving career possibilities for elders			
	Establishing an educational / training fund appropriate to the needs of unskilled workers			
		Wages according to nature of work and personal skill and performance		
	Encourage opportunities for better transfer of workers between different types and fields of work			
Communication		Advertisement / tv-spot campaign to raise age-awareness at the job-market		
		Lectures / counselling / therapy on stress, communication, psychological risk factors etc.		
		Lectures on prevention, communication, corporate culture, social rights etc.		

* *Exercise, nutrition, consumption of alcohol and nicotine, relaxation*

Fig. 10: Summary of actions - Iceland

1. Political basis

Compared to other OECD countries, Iceland has the greatest number of older people in employment. In the age group from 60 to 64 years, Iceland has by far the highest numbers compared to many countries in Europe, as 85 % of individuals in this age group are working (Directorate of Labour - Vinnumálastofnun og Statistics Iceland - Hagstofan). The retirement age among civil employees is 70 and in the private workplaces the most common retirement age is 67. Many employees have the opportunity to retire at an earlier age (60-65 years of age) but may then suffer a decrease in pension payments. Early retirement is therefore not generally a feasible option.

Like other countries in the OECD, Iceland will be facing great social and economic changes in the next decades. A lower birth rate and increased life-span will result in fewer individuals able to work and to contribute to the welfare-system. Nevertheless, health care and pension costs will increase (Report: Ageing and labour markets for older workers, 1999). The Icelandic nation is, therefore, getting older, as are most other European nations, although the increase in age is at a slower rate in Iceland than in many European countries. A report by SA - The Confederation of Icelandic Employers (Samtök atvinnulífsins) - in April 2003, predicts that from the year 2010, the current increase in the number of employees of working age will slow down to about 0.5 % up to the year 2015 vs. 1.0-1.3 % in the year 2000. Given that the economic growth will average 2-3 %, it is therefore clear that the demand for workforce will not be supplied by Icelandic society in the future, given the same development as in recent years.

A survey done by SA - The Confederation of Icelandic Employers (Samtök atvinnulífsins) - in 2002, showed that Icelandic employers value the contributions of older workers as much as those of younger workers. In smaller companies older workers were even considered more valuable than younger staff. Results of another Icelandic survey (Gallup, 2004) do not indicate that older workers are systematically and commonly discriminated on the job market. However, the survey showed that older workers claimed to have fewer opportunities for career advancement. Furthermore, 10 % considered that people at their own workplace had been laid off and/or not re-hired because of age.

The primary role of Administration of Occupational Safety and Health (AOSH) is to prevent accidents and health damage in the workplace. The current legislation, Act on Working Conditions, Health and Safety in the Workplace No. 46/1980, and a number of regulations ratified by the Minister for Social Affairs, cover workplaces on land with a staff of one or more persons. The AOSH is responsible for enforcing the legislation. The core functions of the AOSH are inspection of workplaces, training, publishing and research activities.

1.1. Unemployment

Among those unemployed in the year 2000, 23 % were aged from 60-70 years compared to 36 % in the age group 25-39. However, in the year 2003, of those unemployed, 10 % were between 60-70 years compared to 40 % in the age group 25-39 (Directorate of Labour - Vinnumálastofnun and Statistics Iceland - Hagstofan).

Long-term unemployment rates have increased for all age groups in Iceland over the recent years (Directorate of Labour - Vinnumálastofnun, 2004). In the year 2001, a study was done in the Reykjavik area on the conditions and well being of those who are long-term unemployed. The results of the study showed that long-term unemployment is more common among older workers (over 55) than in other age groups. They were also more likely to claim ill health as a reason for not seeking employment. 11 % of the respondents thought they had been laid off because of age. Also organisational changes and recession were commonly used as reasons, in this age group, for being laid off (Efling - Union, Sólveig Magnúsdóttir, 2001).

1.2. Pension rights and labour market participation

Early retirement is fairly uncommon in Iceland. The reasons are cultural and economic. For decades, there have been low levels of unemployment and a high demand for workforce (Prime Minister´s Office [Forsætisráðuneytið] - Report on flexible retirement, October 2002).

The Icelandic pension system is built on a social security system, mutual insurance/pension funds and personal pension savings. As mentioned earlier the common retirement age is 70 for civil employees and 67 in private workplaces, which is rather high considering data from many other European countries. Entitlement to pension starts at the age of 65. Workers have the option to postpone their retirement until the age of 70. However, civil and municipal workers can retire at the age of 64 and seamen at the age of 60. Social security is funding half of the retirement pension.

The so called "95 year principle" was in practice until 1996. The principle stated that public employees whose biological age plus work age for the state equalled 95 years were entitled to retire. This rule now applies only to those who started working for the state before 1996 but no longer applies after this date. But this group now has the right to work part-time - up to 50 % outside the civil work sector or on an hourly basis within the civil work sector and collect their pension according to the rights they have already acquired.

2. National programmes / projects

2.1. Labour contracts

2.1.1. Private job-market

2.1.1.1. Wage

Individuals' rate of pay is determined by the number of years employed at a company or in a branch. Many union wage-agreements state that employees can transfer their sick leave and pension rights between workplaces.

According to a contract between The Icelandic Confederation of Labour - Alþýðusamband Íslands (ASÍ) - and SA - The Confederation of Icelandic Employers - employers are obliged to give notice long before terminating a job-contract with older workers. Four months' notice has to be given for employees of 55 years and older who have worked consistently in the same company for ten years; five months if the employee is 60 years and six months if the employee is 63 years old. The employee on the other hand is obliged to give three months' notice regardless of age (Source: Summary of basic rights and obligations in the private labour market in Iceland).

2.1.1.2. Training

In 2000, representatives of employers (SA) and employees (ASÍ - The Icelandic Confederation of Labour, VR - The Commercial Workers' Union of Reykjavík) agreed to establish an education/training fund geared to the needs of unskilled workers on the private job-market. The statistics showed that those over fifty years of age were less likely to participate in training projects. In 2003, of those who were funded, 20 % were in the age group from 50-59 years and 15 % in the group of 60+.

Similar agreements have been made between SA and technical trade unions. Also, SA, The Federation of Icelandic Fishing Vessel Owners (Landssamband íslenskra útvegsmanna - LÍÚ) and the Federation of Icelandic Seamen´s Union (Sjómannasamband Íslands - SSÍ) established a training/education fund recently - Sjómennt - starting in autumn 2004.

2.1.2. Civil employees

2.1.2.1. Wage

The most common age group among civil workers is 46-50 (March 2004). Age determines wage-increases for civil employees. General wage-contracts are made but civil/public institutions can agree on special contracts with unions about adjustment to the general wage-contracts according to the needs of institutions and staff. Institutions can, therefore, reward employees based on the nature of work being done and on personal skills and performance.

2.1.2.2. Training

Education/Training funds exist for civil employees in the following trade unions: Association of Academics (Bandalag Háskólamenntaðra manna - BHM), Confederation of State and Municipal Employees (Bandalag starfsmanna ríkis og bæja - BSRB) and The Icelandic Teachers' Union (Kennarasamband Íslands - KÍ).

2.2. Committee on flexible retirement

A committee on flexible retirement working under the Prime Minister's Office conducted a survey about the status of the age group 55-75 on the job-market (Hagfæðistofnun-IMG-Gallup). The study was done in 2002, and results showed that 40 % of study participants in the age group 55-64 wished to decrease working hours at the retirement age of 67 instead of leaving work for good. However, the same percentage of respondents wished to quit working altogether at 67.

2.3. A committee, appointed by the Minister of Social Affairs

was established in February 2004, consisting of different stakeholders, to study the status of middle aged and older workers and also to identify ways to strengthen their position on the job market. Furthermore, the committee was to study whether/in what way legal regulations built on EU Dir. 2000/78 can avert discrimination in terms of age in Icelandic workplaces.

Work done:

- Legal status was studied.
- A survey was done in April-May 2004 on the attitudes towards middle aged and older employees (50-65) on the job market.
- In May 2004, a conference was held with the focus on the issues of middle aged and older workers. It was stressed at the conference that older workers face difficulties in getting new jobs after being laid off or having resigned from previous jobs.
- A report was published in February 2005. The main conclusions of the committee stated in the report were to suggest that the Icelandic government would start a five-year programme to strengthen the position of middle aged and older workers and, furthermore, to ensure that the issues of these group will be publicised and attended to in the coming years.

2.4. An advertisement campaign

A series of television advertisements with the focus on workers aged 50+ was run in June-August 2004 on three Icelandic television channels by VR - The Commercial Workers' Union of Reykjavík. The aim of the advertisement campaign 50+ was to increase awareness of the status of this age group on the job-market and to facilitate positive attitudes amongst employers towards this group.

3. Players

3.1. NGOs / interest group representatives

3.1.1. VR - Verzlunarmarmannafélag Reykjavíkur - The Commercial Workers' Union of Reykjavík

- Has run an advertisement campaign/television advertisements with the focus on workers 50+ from June to August 2004.

- The life span of Icelanders has increased considerably. This development has caused VR to reconsider pension rights and the calculation of pension costs/payments.

3.1.2. SA - Samtök Atvinnulífisins - The Confederation of Icelandic Employers

- SA did a survey on employers' attitudes towards older employees. In the subsequently report, published in 2002, SA indicated that Icelandic employers value the contributions of older workers as much as those of younger workers. In smaller companies the older workers were even considered more valuable than the younger staff.
- A report on ways to improve living conditions of the Icelandic nation was published in April 2003. It suggested that the current increase in number of employees will slow down from the year 2010 on. As the increase in scope of work will slow down the report indicates the importance of increasing the efficiency and flexibility of the workforce so that employees can easily transfer between types of work and different fields of work, such as the public and private sectors.

3.1.3. FEB - Félag eldri borgara - The Federation of Older Citizens

- Interest group for the rights of older and retired individuals.
- Provides counselling and information and give talks on the issues of older workers.

3.2. Research organisations

3.2.1. IMG

IMG is a multinational research and consulting company. Companies in the IMG Group include Gallup Iceland (opinion polls, labour market research, workplace and health and lifestyle research), IMG Deloitte (management consultancy and strategic planning), Management Training and vinna.is, Mannafl and Liðsauki (employment agencies). IMG employs a permanent staff of about 100, over 75 % of whom are university graduates. Alongside the permanent staff, more than 100 people work on data collection and implementation of market surveys and opinion polls.

Surveys done on the issues of older workers include:

- status of the age group 55-75 on the job-market (2004 also in cooperation with Hagfræðistofnun in 2002).

3.2.2. Hagfræðistofnun - Institute of Economic Studies

The institute of economic studies is an independent research institution within the faculty of economics at the University of Iceland. Emphasis is put on competence for the economic analysis of international issues with special emphasis on policy analysis in the following sections:

- growth and development,
- pensions and social security,
- macroeconomic policies,
- energy economics,
- resource economics, and
- risk and financial markets.

Surveys done on the issues of older workers include:

- status of the age group 55-75 on the job-market (in cooperation with IMG-Gallup in 2002).

No suggestions on special measures for an ageing workforce were given in the two studies by IMG and IMG/Hagfræðistofnun.

3.2.3. Research Centre for Occupational Health and Working Life

The research centre conducts multidisciplinary research and gives lectures on health and safety for employees, including older workers. The centre is a cooperation project between the University of Iceland and the Administration of Occupational Safety and Health. No special approaches were yet followed but all data was analysed and studied in terms of different age groups at workplaces.

4. Projects

4.1. Landsbankinn - The National Bank of Iceland

The bank employs 1,500 individuals. The programme "Retirement - New Future" prepares employees who are soon to retire for this change in their life. It also provides necessary information about pension rights, taxes and how to deal with their spare time. Methods used are lectures, conversations and training, with the emphasis on the participation of employees. This program was chosen as a model of best practice in a project of European Mental Health Promotion and Prevention strategy in Europe 2001-2003.

Aims of the project:

- Preparing the target group for the changes corresponding with retirement.
- Broadening the overall perspective and personal view.
- Increasing the level of well being after retirement and educating prospective retirees about various issues (family, finances, time, physical and psychological issues) and decreasing possible anxiety connected with retirement.

Landsbankinn does not put any emphasis on keeping employees at work longer - because of the high retirement age - but it tries to make the transition to retirement easier for its employees.

4.2. Islandsbanki - ISB

The bank employs 950 individuals. ISB prepares employees for retirement via educational training courses with various specialists, focusing on different issues such as pension and social security rights, finance, health and exercise. Furthermore, specialists in geriatric medicine give talks in the courses; counselling regarding social rights is offered. People can attend these courses twice, that is, two years before retirement and again at retirement age. Employees at the bank can choose whether they retire between the age of 65 or 67 years. Islandsbanki offers social programmes for retired employees. Emphasis is laid on mixing education and fun. Educational meetings are held, courses are given and trips are taken. Retired employees have, furthermore, access to summerhouses owned by the employee-association of the bank.

Ireland

Nadia Clarkin, Richard Wynne

<table>
<tr><th>Field of promotion</th><th>Physical strain</th><th>Psyche / cognition</th><th>Mental / social competence</th><th>Professional competence</th></tr>
<tr><td>Action</td><td colspan="4"></td></tr>
<tr><td>Relief of physical strain / WHP actions</td><td colspan="2">Setting-based measures</td><td></td><td></td></tr>
<tr><td></td><td colspan="2">Behaviour-based measures *</td><td></td><td></td></tr>
<tr><td></td><td colspan="3">Monitoring and enforcing compliance with OSH legislation</td><td></td></tr>
<tr><td></td><td colspan="4">Age diversity management</td></tr>
<tr><td>Age-related working hours</td><td colspan="3">Adoption of family friendly work practices</td><td></td></tr>
<tr><td></td><td colspan="4">Job-sharing</td></tr>
<tr><td></td><td colspan="3">Part-time working</td><td></td></tr>
<tr><td></td><td colspan="3">Gradual reduction of working time before retirement</td><td></td></tr>
<tr><td></td><td colspan="3">Flexible system of retirement</td><td></td></tr>
<tr><td>Qualification</td><td colspan="4">Lifelong learning</td></tr>
<tr><td></td><td></td><td colspan="3">Training the trainer</td></tr>
<tr><td></td><td colspan="4">Skill development for older workers (IT, service, communication, customers relation)</td></tr>
<tr><td></td><td colspan="4">Strategic recruitment and retention of older workers</td></tr>
<tr><td>Communication</td><td></td><td colspan="3">Raising awareness on lifestyle issues</td></tr>
<tr><td></td><td colspan="3">Work-life balance - a guideline</td><td></td></tr>
<tr><td></td><td colspan="4">Age profile analysis</td></tr>
</table>

Field of promotion	Physical strain	Psyche / cognition	Mental / social competence	Professional competence
	Staff opinion survey			
	Organising a best practice study visit			
	Establishing an all island network for WHP			
	National Health Promotion Co-ordinator (planned) for advising on implementation of WHP measures			
	Publishing guidelines of equality and diversity training and on equality policies			
	Pilot training programmes for managers, supervisors and older workers			
	Publishing research on workplace hazards and risks			
	Audit HR policies and disseminate revised policies			
	Establishing a steering group and develop pilot programmes (review and action plan inclusive)			

** Exercise, nutrition, consumption of alcohol and nicotine, relaxation*

Fig. 11: Summary of actions - Ireland

By the year 2011 it is estimated that persons aged 65 and over will represent 14.1 per cent of the Irish Republic's population and persons in the 45-69-year old category will have increased by 24 %. It has been suggested that by 2050 there will be 40 people aged over 65 for every 100 working people. This presents a major challenge for the Irish labour market.

In Ireland, there are a number of health focused and other initiatives targeting older people in general. However, it appears that there are few initiatives specifically targeting older people in employment. This situation arises in the Irish context as Ireland lags behind the rest of Europe in terms of the age profile of its workers and older workers do not present a major issue in the short term. In this regard some recent policy has begun to consider the issue of older workers; however, as yet there appears to be very little specifically dealing with workplace health promotion for this target group. Also awareness raising of the issue of older workers more generally has begun to take place at national level.

1. Political basis

1.1. Health and Safety at Work Act 1989

Although the body of legislation is seen as broadly supportive of workplace health promotion, there is very little evidence that it has played any role in promoting activities which go beyond statutory responsibilities. Furthermore, there is some evidence pointing out that even "traditional" health and safety activities are not applied universally, and this is particularly the case for the SME sector.
Government of Ireland (1989) Health and Safety Act. Dublin, Stationery Office

1.2. Employment Equality Act 1998

The purpose of this Act is to make provision for the promotion of equality between employed persons and to outlaw discrimination in relation to employment. The scope of the Act is comprehensive and prohibits direct and indirect discrimination, victimisation, dismissal, harassment and sexual harassment on nine grounds:

- gender
- marital status
- family status
- sexual orientation
- religion
- age (18-65 years of age)
- disability
- race
- membership of the travelling community

Government of Ireland (1998) Employment Equality Act. Dublin, Stationery Office

With the Employment Equality Act (1998) wide-ranging protections against age discrimination in recruitment, dismissals and training were established in Irish law for the first time. Under this Act, all aspects of employment are covered, e.g. equal pay/remuneration, access to employment, vocational training, conditions of employment (including overtime, shift-work etc.), training or experience.

The law includes a provision that allows positive action to be taken to recruit more employees aged over 50. Unfortunately, the Act has an upper age limit of 65 for its operation - which means that people over 65 who experience discrimination at work are not protected by its terms.

The statutory remit of working towards the elimination of discrimination and of promoting equal opportunities at work comes up to the Equality Authority established under the Employment Equality Act. It provides information and gives advice to the public on the operation of this Act and other relevant pieces of legislation.

1.3. Equal Status Acts 2000 and 2004

In 2000, the *Equal Status Act* came into operation. This law sought to promote equality, prohibit certain kinds of discrimination and prohibit harassment. In effect, the law extended the ban on discrimination to anybody buying goods, using services, obtaining accommodation and attending educational establishments on the same nine grounds as the *Employment Equality Act*, including age.

One significant difference between the two pieces of legislation is that the upper age limit of 65 does not apply in the *Equal Status Act.*

The Act was updated in 2004 given the necessity to implement the employment and non-employment aspects of the Race Directive (2000/43/EC), the Framework Employment Directive (2000/78/EC) and the Gender Equal Treatment Directive (2002/73/EC). It also provides for a number of procedural amendments to the Employment Equality Act 1998 and the Equal Status Act 2000.B.

Government of Ireland (2000) Equal Status Act. Dublin, Stationery Office
Government of Ireland (2004) Equal Status Act. Dublin, Stationery Office

2. National programmes / projects

2.1. EQUAL Project - National Flexi-work Partnership

Project Aim

The aim of this project is to develop new models of working which will:

- facilitate the reconciliation of work and family life,
- include groups that have hitherto had difficulty in attaining or maintaining employment, and
- encourage employers and policy makers to incorporate these models into their normal practices.

Project Objectives

- To gain a fuller understanding of the needs of the target groups through research;
- to stimulate the development of innovative pilot schemes involving family friendly policies;
- to utilise the experience of companies with greater experience of flexible working arrangements to promote these policies in other workplaces;
- to encourage the maintenance in employment of groups of workers who have been excluded by virtue of stigma as well as inflexible working patterns;

- to produce guidelines for employers on employing people with mental health difficulties and guidelines for employers on employing older people, and
- to facilitate the incorporation of these innovative models into standard mainstream practice.

Project Actions

- *Research*
  This will involve a nationwide representative survey of 1,000 people to ascertain their current conditions, needs and aspirations in relation to work and quality of life. There will be a particular focus on people with mental health needs and older people, with an additional sample of 200 of each.
- *Pilot Project 3* looks specifically at "flexible forms of working for older workers" and will produce "Guidelines for Employers on Employing Older People" in conjunction with IBEC (see 3.2.3.).

During this project a number of pilot projects aimed at retaining or getting older people back into work through more flexible work measures will be identified and run. So far an initiative called "Term time for grandparents" has been implemented and is yet to be evaluated. Findings from these pilots will be available later in 2005.

Products

- Final research report,
- summary report,
- guidelines regarding employment of target groups,
- conferences - academic community, employers, employees, and
- research reports for academic community.

Equal projects - National Flexi-work Partnership at (http://www.equal-ci.ie/2000/proj/flexi.html)

2.2. Implementing equality for older people report by Equality Authority

In June 2002, the Equality Authority published a report, "Implementing Equality for Older People in Ireland". This report seeks to examine and expose the issue of ageism and to put forward an equality agenda with a capacity to change the situation and experience of older people in our society. Age & Opportunity and other ageing organisations were represented on the advisory committee to the report. The report has a chapter on working which looks at access to work, employment options, barriers to work, retirement options, unemployment, pensions and work-life balance for older workers (over 50 years old). It also makes recommendations regarding the use of positive action measures in the return to work of older workers. It also recommends that the Department of Trade, Enterprise and Employment and FÁS (state training authority) undertake actions such as targeted training and returning older workers to work.
Implementing Equality for Older People (2002) Equality Authority, Dublin: Equality Authority.

2.3. Adding Years to Life and Life to Years: A Health Promotion strategy for Older People. (NCAOP)

"Adding Years to Life and Life to Years: A Health Promotion Strategy for Older People" was produced by the Council in 1998 in association with the Department of Health and Children, marking the launch of the Council's Healthy Ageing Programme. It complements existing national health strategies including the National Cancer Strategy and the National Alcohol Policy.

The Strategy analyses life expectancy and illness figures, lifestyle and behaviour trends among older people in Ireland. It sets out national goals and targets for improving the health and well-being of older people and proposes recommended action plans at national and local levels.

The aims of the Healthy Ageing Programme are:

- to improve life expectancy at age 65 and beyond,
- to improve the health status of people age 65 and beyond,
- to improve the lives and autonomy of older people who are already affected by illness and impairment, and

- to increase the expectation of a healthy and enjoyable old age.

The Programme aims to support a range of sectors with a role to play in healthy ageing through development and capacity-building in the areas of networking, training, materials, models of good practice, national partnership initiatives, public awareness and evaluation of initiatives.

Current areas of activity:

- Healthy Ageing Database and Report,
- Directory of Healthy Ageing Information Resources for Older People, and
- research.

It addresses health promotion for older people in its broadest sense, acknowledging the impact of environmental and social factors such as housing, security, transport, attitudes and income on the quality of life of older people.
Adding years to life and life to years - NCAOP at
http://www.ncaop.ie/publications/research/factfiles/FF14Accidents.pdf

3. Players

European Foundation on Working and Living Conditions

A study done in late 1990s looked at retention, retraining and reintegration of older workers. The output was a good practice guide with portfolio of 150 initiatives - unfortunately Ireland was not represented amongst the case studies. New research planned for 2005 will be looking at age management in the workplace - output of which is due at the end of that year. This is a 10 country study and Ireland is not participating again. The title of this project is Employment Initiatives for an Ageing Workforce. A few examples will look at WHP, the majority will be HR related.

3.1. State

3.1.1. Department of Health

The Department of Health established a Health Promotion Unit in 1988. The main functions of this unit are policy development, research and evaluation, also to raise awareness of lifestyle issues through multi-media information campaigns and the development of relevant materials for the public.

In 1999, the Health Promotion Unit published the policy document "Healthy bodies - healthy work", which outlined the need to adopt a proactive approach in the workplace setting. The issue of Workplace Health Promotion has since been developed and expanded within each of the eight Health Boards in the state appointing a Workplace Coordinator. The Workplace Coordinator has the responsibility for the development of workplace health promotion plans and the initiation of pilot projects at regional level. At present, there are no systematic or strategic Workplace Health Promotion initiatives targeted at directly older workers through this structure. However, Workplace Coordinators mentioned that at local level there may well be programmes initiated by interested parties on an ad hoc basis which consider issues more pertinent to older workers (e.g. osteoporosis).

More recently a number of work-related initiatives have been outlined in the National Health Promotion Strategy 2000-2005. These include plans for the appointment of a National Workplace Health Promotion Coordinator, the examination of the needs of small to medium-seized enterprises in relation to workplace health promotion and the continued implementation of the cardiovascular strategies in the workplace setting. The coordinator will also be in a position to advise on the development of best practice in implementing workplace health initiatives both at national and regional levels.

To further support and expand this initiative, the Health Promotion Unit has established an all island network for Workplace Health Promotion which has met twice to date. Members include the Health and Safety Authority. The Network recognises the need for a multi-sectoral approach involving other statutory and non-statutory agencies, stakeholders involved and the social partners to tackle workplace health issues and to support the implementation and evaluation of current workplace health promotion programmes. (http://www.healthpromotion.ie/health_promotion_strategy/)

3.1.2. Health and Safety Authority

The Health and Safety Authority is the national body in Ireland charged with responsibility for securing health and safety at work. It is a state-sponsored body, established under the Safety, Health and Welfare at Work Act (1989), and it operates under the aegis of the Department of Enterprise, Trade and Employment.

The Authority's primary functions are to:

- monitor and enforce compliance with occupational health and safety legislation,
- provide information and expert advice to employers, employees and the self-employed,
- promote workplace safety, health, welfare, education and training,
- publish research on workplace hazards and risks, and
- to propose new regulations and codes of practice to the Minister.

The Health and Safety Authority (HSA) is largely preoccupied with traditional, mainstream activities. This is attributed to the resources constraint (mainly staff) and the agency opted to prioritise high-risk sectors (construction and agriculture) instead.

3.1.3. Equality Authority

The Equality Authority was established in 1999 to work towards the elimination of discrimination in employment, and in the provision of goods and services, education, property and other opportunities to which the public generally have access. It provides information, advice and support for equal opportunities. The Authority has an in-house legal service and provides a free confidential information and advisory service. If a person has a query or a complaint regarding employment discrimination on grounds of age, for example, they can direct their complaint to the Equality Authority.

Equality Authority convened the Equal Opportunities Framework Committee with the social partners: publishing guidelines of equality and diversity training and on equality policies to support planned and systematic approaches to workplace equality, and providing funding to a range of projects.

A co-funded Equality Studies Unit has been established in the Equality Authority under the Employment and Human Resources Development Operation Programme (EHRDOP) to support the integration of people with disabilities, refugees, travellers and older people into the labour market.

The unit will pursue three priorities:

- to improve information and monitoring of the situation in relation to the above named categories,
- examine the application of the equal opportunities principle in selected measures, and
- to disseminate research findings and develop practical resource materials for providers.

3.1.4. Department of Enterprise, Trade and Employment

The National Employment Action Plan of the Department of Enterprise, Trade and Employment covers the period 2003-2005, and is set against a much-changed economic background. The global economic environment has changed and the challenge for Ireland over the coming years is to consolidate its achievements and to maintain low levels of unemployment.

The priority areas for employment policy as outlined in the Plan are:

- more emphasis on R&D investment,
- greater regional spread of investment,
- firms taking greater responsibility for up-skilling their employees,
- lifelong learning,
- adoption of family friendly work practices, and
- support for disadvantaged people to take up employment.

The plan makes reference to older workers in two main ways. Through FÁS Ireland, it is participating in the OECD thematic review of policies to improve labour market outcomes for older workers. The Department intends to review how older people can extend their working life without being financially or socially penalised and will seek to remove financial disincentives and the requirement on those aged 55-66 to retire in order to qualify for pensions.

To this end, increases of over 20 % in the income tax exemption limits for those aged 65 and over were introduced in the 2002 Budget. Also, the Back-To-Work Allowance has been re-focused in favour of longer term and older unemployed people.
(http://www.entemp.ie/)

3.1.5. FÁS (Foras Áiseanna Saothair - Training & Employment Authority)

FÁS, Ireland's National Training and Employment Authority, was established in January 1988, under the Labour Services Act 1987, to provide a wide range of services to the labour market in Ireland. It provides training and retraining, apprenticeships, recruitment service, employment schemes and assistance to community groups and advice to people returning to Ireland and those seeking employment elsewhere in the EU.

One of the Employment Schemes - the Community Employment Scheme - has a section dealing with New Flexibility for Older Workers and other participants. This covers individuals who continue to experience difficulties in getting jobs following their participation on CE Schemes. Difficulties usually arise due to age, health, literacy, numeracy problems or a lack of suitable jobs locally. In recognition of this, the three-year limit on participation for people over 50 years of age has been removed for those people over 50 who, having spent three years on the Programme continue to experience difficulties in getting employment. For such participants FÁS will have discretion, within limits, to offer a further period on the Programme on a case by case basis.
(www.fas.ie)

3.1.6. National Economic and Social Forum

The functions of the Forum is to advise the government on policies to achieve greater equality and social inclusion, and such other matters as may be specified by the government in the context of social partnership arrangements, by analysing, monitoring and evaluating relevant programmes and policies.

A recent report - "Labour market issues for older workers", Forum Report No. 26, February 2003 - focuses on measures to retain and enhance the participation of older workers, as well as the unemployed or those discouraged from seeking work and older women who have not been in paid work for a long time. The key concept underpinning the discussion in the report is that of choice.

Older workers should have a greater degree of choice about when to retire, about flexible working arrangements and a more supportive working environment with access to better training and progression. It proposed that for this purpose, current policies and employment practices will have to be

adapted so that older workers are more effectively supported by employers and by society generally.
Labour market issues for older workers (2003). Forum Report No. 26 National Economic Social Forum. Dublin, Ireland.

3.2. NGOs / interest groups representatives

3.2.1. Chambers of Commerce of Ireland (CCI)

In response to the growing proportion of older people in Ireland, CCI has established the ARROW (Assisting the Recruitment & Retention of Older Workers) network, which assists companies specifically with the recruitment and retention of older workers. The ARROW programme aims to break down the perceptual barriers and focus on the value of strategically recruiting older workers. It covers practicalities around company performance and the employment, training, motivation, and strategic recruitment of older workers. To date, CCI has:

- developed and delivered pilot training programmes for managers, supervisors and older workers,
- developed a network of companies within the greater Dublin region with specific interest in older workers,
- held a number of network and information seminars, and
- organised a best practice study visit for member companies to a networking conference in Vienna on Managing an Ageing Workforce.

The programme takes a hands-on approach to the skills development of older workers by training older workers in practical work skills including IT skills, customer service skills and communication, and focuses on ensuring that their skills are up to date and they are as flexible in what they can do as younger staff. The training cost is heavily subsidised by the Skillnets training initiative. The training programmes developed to date as part of the programme include:

Level 1: HR Managers/SME Owner Managers

- Strategic Recruitment and Retention of Older Workers
- Understanding Pensions & Reward Issues for Older Workers
- Equality Legislation & Best Practice Employment of Older Workers

- EU Legislation with regard to Age
- Employment Law Update
- Case Studies in Age Equality

Level 2: Managers & Supervisors
- Diversity in the Workplace
- Train the Trainer
- Interviewing Techniques: Keeping Within the Law

Level 3: Older Workers
- Winning the Customer
- Communications
- Excellence Through Sales
- Occupational Health and Safety Training: Combating Stress
- Occupational Health and Safety Training: Food Safety
- Occupational Health and Safety Training: Manual Handling
- Occupational First Aid
- IT Skills

Going forward it is planned to expand the network both within Dublin, and to set up regional networks of companies through local chambers. (http://www.chambers.ie)

3.2.2. NCAOP

This umbrella body has an extensive database of all projects/initiatives, which target older people in general; however, initiatives exclusively for older workers and health promotion are not a feature of this database.

With regard to older people working the NCAOP suggests that a more flexible system of retirement which could include phased retirement, involving a gradual reduction in the number or hours, days, or weeks worked in the years before complete retirement would be a useful measure to maintain older workers in the workplace. Also important would be an increase in the availability of part-time work or job-sharing positions and an alteration in the accepted time of retirement. This would allow individuals the choice of retirement at any time between certain fixed points (e.g. 60 to 70 years of age).

3.2.3. Irish Business and Employers Confederation (IBEC)

IBEC represents the interests of businesses and employers by shaping policies and influencing decision-making.

In 2003, IBEC produced a guide on employment of older workers. This guide provides practical advice to employers on introducing age diversity strategy in their organisations and on attracting and retaining older workers. This is the first guideline to focus exclusively on older people in the Irish workplace and is a response to the anticipated ageing population.

Developed by IBEC in association with the National Flexi-Work Partnership, the guideline is supported by AGE Action Ireland, Trinity College, FÁS, and ICTU and AWARE. It is based on experiences drawn from IBEC's involvement in projects with organisations representing the needs of older people in Ireland as well as IBEC's counterpart organisations in Germany, Denmark and the Netherlands.

The guideline urges employers to take six strategic steps, which IBEC believes will achieve an age diverse workplace that reflects the diversity of the population. The steps are:

1) compose an equal opportunities statement and policy,
2) carry out an age profile analysis,
3) conduct a staff opinion survey,
4) audit HR policies and disseminate revised policies,
5) establish a steering group and develop a pilot programme, and
6) review the pilot programme and develop an action plan.

The publication of the Guideline coincided with IBEC's third Work-Life Balance National Roundtable entitled, "Work-Life Balance - Everybody's Business". Research shows that providing flexible working options is an effective inducement to older workers.

3.3. Private / commercial service enterprises

none

3.4. Research organisations

none

4. Projects

The authors have not been able to identify any WHP initiatives which specifically target the group of older workers.

There would appear to be a number of reasons for this lack of activity:

- Ireland has the youngest workforce in Europe and consequently there is relatively little emphasis on the issue of older workers, either by policy makers or by workplace health professionals.
- Employment rates amongst older workers are very high by EU standards (more than 40 % of 60-65-year-olds are in employment - by contrast, the EU average is about 30 %).
- Levels of disability, as measured by the numbers of disability pensions, are low and most people on disability pensions are older workers. As a result, there is not the pressure on policies or services to target older workers.
- Levels of workplace health promotion are relatively low. The policy support and the service infrastructure needed to implement workplace health promotion on a widespread scale are lacking in Ireland.

Italy

Lamberto Briziarelli, Giuseppe Masanotti, Sergio Perticaroli

Field of promotion	Physical strain	Psyche / cognition	Mental / social competence	Professional competence
Action				
Relief of physical strain / WHP actions				
Age-related working hours	Part-time jobs for aged			
Qualification	Craftsman training for aged			
	Promotion of training facilities			
	"The Elderly to Work" - training young people			
Communication	Promotion of corporate social responsibility			

Fig. 12: Summary of actions - Italy

1. Political basis

The *Italian Constitution*, adopted on December 22, 1947, effective since January 1, 1948, contains the principles and gives the legal basis for all laws in Italy. No laws, especially in the field of health and, in particular, in the field of occupational health, ever questioned the principle of guaranteeing health for all Italians.

Italian policy promotes the social cohesion of its society especially through encouraging measures for families and households which takes care for the elders in their families. It also makes way to the change from a *welfare-state* to a *welfare-community*.

Ministry of Welfare (Ministry of Labour and Social Affairs)

White paper proposals for a welfare system in a dynamic and solitary society, Rome, February 2003.

The purpose of this White Paper is to outline a reference framework for the attainment and enhancement of social cohesion in Italy. Special emphasis is put on the demographic transition and its effects on intergenerational relations and on the family services.

2. National programmes / projects

2.1. Communication

In accordance with the afore mentioned White Paper, national programmes in several regions and municipalities offer services for the ageing at local level: part-time jobs (social jobs for the community), craftsman training etc. Three initiatives may serve as examples:

- *Internet Saloon for the elderly: a positive experience*

A big software developer together with AIM (a Milanese non profit association) has set up an Internet Saloon: a site to teach older people the advantages that they could derive from the use of the new technologies.

It started on October 2, 2000, and provides courses at eighteen computer terminals connected to Internet. After the first year 3,000 participants had qualified as "senior navigators". The software company has decided to continue the initiative in other Italian cities in collaboration with local governments and associations.

• *Grandparent on Internet 2003 - 2nd edition*

The Consortium Digital Youth, again with the contribution of a software developer, promoted the second edition of "Grandparent on Internet". The initiative, active from October to December 2003, took place in Rome, where elders and students of the University of Rome worked together. The approach was that the students acted as trainers for the "grandparents", occasionally assisted by a teacher experienced in new technologies.

• *Piazze Telematiche*

An initiative very closely related to the one already mentioned was initially exclusively financed by the European Commission. More details can be found on these websites: www.comune.napoli.it and www.piazzetelematiche.it

2.2. The areas of intervention

Italian politics consider the family to be an active subject and give it a leading role in the organisation of the welfare system. There are two further considerations here.

Firstly - as well as their unchanged role of solving a variety of crucial social situations - social policies have to develop their preventive function to a greater extent. This applies in particular to all those situations linked to living and working conditions.

The *second* point is that the social policies should not only address people's public health demands but they also have to cover a large spectrum of problems ranging from social integration, intergenerational coherence to the development of solidarity networks - characteristics peculiar to societies and communities based on sharing and solidarity.

This new approach incorporates the new EU policy guidelines in full, whether included in the European Charter of Fundamental Rights or resulting from the Lisbon European Council.

2.2.1. The right to universal services through a new solidarity

For individuals or families who run the risk of exclusion from special services a guaranteed right of access to a "universal service" (primary social services and primary services in a broader sense) is aimed at. To achieve this goal, institutional actors at various governance levels, households, family associations, volunteer associations etc. will be integrated. Even the further development of formal and informal solidarity networks has been reconsidered.

First achievements have been made by the definition of a new normative framework for improved access to social services. Within a liberalised economic interrelationship, access to social services for the disadvantaged has to be guaranteed.

The primary objective is the creation, interaction and integration of solidarity networks, e.g. mutual family aid networks. In cooperation with already existing actors of the primary social sector - public or private - technical innovations should also be integrated, and training facilities for actors and users of the services are to be promoted. So far there are no national agreements but local initiatives on network level (school, municipality, SME, trade unions) are supported. Thus any resulting action is focused even more on local communities and their resources.

The current process defines essential levels of social services together with regional and local authorities; territorial differences and thus different starting points are taken into account. There has to be a basis to define a grid for the areas of intervention, the types of services and benefits to be provided. Innovative guidelines for necessary interventions and services have to be implemented.

2.2.2. Social inclusion

The implementation of measures for social inclusion is the responsibility of institutional agencies at various levels; third sector and volunteer associations as well as households.

Priority is given to social integration and work placement of individuals at risk of exclusion. The most common poverty traps may be identified through situations resulting from unemployment or particular social vulnerability. By defining appropriate measures it might be possible to evade poverty.

Taxation, employment, education, housing policy and social health are the fields where actions would have the best effect.

Thus, an effective income policy is the major tool to

- give stability and strength to economic growth,
- ensure a continuing balance of public finances consistent with the commitments of the stability and growth pact defined in the Europcan Council at Seville,

- safeguard the purchasing power of wages, and
- attain an increase in the employment rate and reduce social exclusion, in accordance with the decision of the European Council in Lisbon.

The tax reform of the 2003 Budget law (Legge Finanziaria) points towards tax-reduction for individuals, households and enterprises and aims at economic development, stimulating consumption and growth.

Since 2003, the income supporting system - "Minimum Placement Income" - has been supplemented by an instrument of the last instance. It is characterised by solidarity-based elements and financed through general taxation. The "Minimum Placement Income" prevents individuals from being singled out through legal and centralistic criteria when entitling them to enter this social security network.

Steps are taken to find out the financial needs of those who are unemployed (to be dealt with by active labour policies which avoid the creation of chronic attitudes and welfare dependency) as well as requirements typical for social vulnerability usually requiring social and income-support measures.

Regarding the employment of young people and individuals facing a high risk of exclusion from the labour market (disabled persons, older adults lacking the required occupational skills etc.) a comprehensive action programme focusing on the integration of vulnerable persons is presently being implemented. The main focus is on the system of education and training when integrating such persons into the labour market. This action program has been worked out in close cooperation with the regions with recourse to the European Social Fund.

2.2.3. Psychophysical autonomy

Individuals suffering from physical and/or mental disabilities, senile motor-type dependence, chronic diseases (Alzheimer's disease) and the like, as well as their families, need the special attention of society. The aim of this action is to guarantee access to employment and assistance for all those individuals suffering from serious limitations to their physical and psychological autonomy. Institutional agencies at various levels, families and their associations, the world of work, and social partners should become involved in these actions.

Until now the Italian social health system has been unable to provide these persons with sufficient health care and social services. Therefore the 2003 action plan - in a coordinated effort of the Ministries of Labour and Social Affairs and of Health - stipulates actions aimed at this group. The possibility for persons affected to stay within their families and in their social environment, the preservation and, as far as possible, the recovery of their personal autonomy and the creation of special territorial services are objectives. The action plan has become operational in an experimental form in a few regions that were willing to contribute in co-financing and organising. No further details are known so far.

2.2.4. The social cohesion of the communities

One main objective of Italian social policy is to promote the social cohesion of individuals and households through the setting up of networks. They should - on the one hand - be capable of raising intergenerational solidarity and - on the other hand - of promoting the inclusion of individuals and groups at risk of exclusion. This should especially be true for marginal communities (i.e. the homeless), communities of legal immigrants with integration difficulties, or elderly persons living on their own.

A special role in developing formal and informal solidarity networks is assigned to household-based initiatives. As coexistence among the generations leads to a mutually enriching social exchange, a new housing policy should be aimed for.

Furthermore, the government should actively back up a couple's decision to have children as well as to accept responsibility for persons who are partially or not fully self-sufficient within their own family networks. The implementation of the Family-Network Monitoring Centre can serve as a useful example.

The setting up of a network comprising 25 municipalities (one per region, two in the most densely populated regions), experts, representatives of regions, provinces and municipalities, as well as representatives of family associations helps to strengthen the cooperation among the agencies working in this sector. This allows existing information and experience to become common knowledge. The monitoring centre, established within the Bologna Municipality, became operational in June 2003, and is financed by resources of the Fund for Social Policies.

With reference to the policies of the volunteer associations, a study scheduled to begin in 2003, should have led to the formulation of a hypothesis for the review of regulations governing the different aspects of social cohesion. No details are known so far.

2.2.5. Corporate Social Responsibility (CSR)

The Italian project promoting corporate social responsibility (CSR) applies also to small and medium-sized enterprises that are traditionally an integral part of local communities. The Government is devoted to making enterprises more aware of the benefits that may be gained from cooperation among institutions, businesses and different sectors of society.

In order to attain these goals, dialogue with the social partners and the civil society has to be strengthened and promotion of CSR instruments and practices has to be enhanced. Exchange of information and best practices has to be integrated in Italian management schemes.

The goals to be attained are as follows:

- to work out a simple and modular social standard for social responsibility which can be applied voluntarily by enterprises,
- to arrange suitable measurements for gaining an insight into and evaluating the social performance of enterprises while regarding tax paying capacities, and
- to contribute to the dissemination of corporate social responsibility culture among enterprises.

3. Players

All institutional players act at various levels, in the private sector and in volunteer associations.

4. Projects

For the moment no relevant WHP projects in companies have been found, therefore two local programmes are cited:

Several regions (Friuli Venezia Giulia, Emilia Romagna, Lombardy), enacting regional laws, have promoted incentives for those enterprises that take on people who have been out of work for more than 12-24 months and are older than 40 years. Also several provinces, Bergamo (see below), Bologna and Verona have organised their offices to offer free training in different fields.

4.1. Bergamo Province - Reintroducing persons over 40 into the job market

Anyone older than 40-45 years, regardless of experience or profession, is in particular difficulty on a dynamic job market, especially if they are women or have no high-school degree.

Measures adopted till now - in reorientation and training - have been important and effective, but new investments have become crucial: it is necessary to evaluate the proposed actions (often unknown), to promote well elaborated interventions, and to support those people expelled from the market who now intend to get back in.

The programme intends to:

- define the category of the over 40-year-olds in more detail and include these details in the data bank; better information on the "expelled" workers, who are very often from small enterprises and who aren't attractive for reemployment,
- to increase the competences of the public operators in the centres for employment,
- take initiatives for the reintroduction in the job market: tutors will guide the applicants (orientation, budget of competences, retraining - not only on new production processes or technology, but also on stress etc. - stage and apprenticeships), and
- involve enterprises in order to find the necessary tools directed to prevent the professional ageing of their employees.

4.2. Municipality of Battipaglia (Salerno)

The project is aimed at the integration of the elderly in the town's society, which is why the municipality of Battibaglia (SA) decided to promote the project, entitled "The elderly to work". It is something between volunteering and work. The initiative aims to involve the elderly in activities which benefit the public in general. The participants take on small jobs near/in the libraries and public/private offices, watch over the safety of children going in and out of school, take care of the city parks, and above all they participate in training activities for the young in order to prevent old arts and handicraft activities from being forgotten. Every participant involved is paid on a hourly basis.

Luxembourg

Paul Weber

<table>
<tr><th>Field of promotion</th><th>Physical strain</th><th>Psyche / cognition</th><th>Mental / social competence</th><th>Professional competence</th></tr>
<tr><td>Action</td><td colspan="4"></td></tr>
<tr><td>Relief of physical strain / WHP actions</td><td colspan="2">WHP actions *</td><td></td><td></td></tr>
<tr><td></td><td colspan="2">Improve working conditions</td><td></td><td></td></tr>
<tr><td></td><td colspan="4">Develop monitor post for seniors</td></tr>
<tr><td></td><td colspan="4">Audits and advisory duties suited the skills of older workers</td></tr>
<tr><td>Age-related working hours</td><td colspan="2">No night shifts for seniors</td><td></td><td></td></tr>
<tr><td></td><td colspan="3">Improve opportunities for part time work, more flexible regulations</td><td></td></tr>
<tr><td></td><td colspan="2">Introduce gradual pre-retirement</td><td></td><td></td></tr>
<tr><td></td><td colspan="2">Reform early retirement schemes</td><td></td><td></td></tr>
<tr><td>Qualification</td><td></td><td colspan="3">Provide more vocational training - encourage through financial incentives</td></tr>
<tr><td></td><td></td><td colspan="3">Promote personal development</td></tr>
<tr><td></td><td colspan="4">Increase job interest</td></tr>
<tr><td></td><td colspan="4">Better career prospects, possibly start a second career</td></tr>
<tr><td></td><td colspan="4">Promote the validation and recognition of working experience</td></tr>
<tr><td></td><td colspan="4">Develop systems to recognise, certify and validate experience gained at the job</td></tr>
<tr><td>Communication</td><td colspan="4">Age-friendly HR policy</td></tr>
<tr><td></td><td colspan="4">National campaign to change attitudes toward seniors</td></tr>
</table>

Field of promotion	Physical strain	Psyche / cognition	Mental / social competence	Professional competence
	Raise awareness at workplaces towards age-related discrimination			
	Internet site for MOGP			
	Database on older workers to analyse and target priority categories			
	Keep individuals informed regularly on their pension entitlement			

** Exercise, nutrition, consumption of alcohol and nicotine, relaxation*

Fig. 13: Summary of actions - Luxembourg

1. Political basis

1.1. Preconditions

Luxembourg has a very special position within the EC.

Being a very small country, Luxembourg has a very large foreign population and an economy that relies heavily on the cross-border labour market. Due to Luxembourg's ability to attract large numbers of foreigners and thus tapping the labour pool of neighbouring regions, little impact of the ageing of its resident population has been experienced so far.

However, this situation might deteriorate in the coming decades. Assuming that the current demographic trends based on highly positive net migration continue, the ratio of population over 65 to the population aged 20-64 would be 40 % in 2050, as compared to slightly under one quarter in 2000.

If demographic trends are assumed to be less favourable with a gradual decline in the number of foreigners entering the country, there would be a stagnation of the resident population, including the foreign population. In this case, in 2050 the population over 65 would be equal to 52 % of the population in the 20-64 age group.

In any event, it is very likely that substantial income transfers will be required from future generations of workers to meet the additional cost of pensions. At present, the contributions of cross-border workers serve to maintain a surplus in the pension funds, but the viability of the pension system is not guaranteed in the long term.

Jobs in Luxembourg remain very attractive to immigrants as well as to cross-border workers because of high salaries and excellent social benefits. The public sector, however, which virtually only recruits Luxembourg nationals - one of the conditions for employment is mastery of three languages, Luxembourgish, German and French - might soon be facing the ageing of its staff and hence a shortage of skilled labour.

The growing imbalance between retired and employed persons could be partially offset by an active policy to encourage women and workers over the age of 50 to remain in employment or return to work. Luxembourg is a country where workers leave the labour market early: the average effective retirement age during the 1997-2002 period was estimated at 59.8 for men and women which is among the lowest in OECD countries.

1.2. The current situation: early retirement of workers over the age of 50

For over two decades, Luxembourg has been promoting the withdrawal of older workers from the labour market through public policies and corporate practices. Numerous, relatively generous, early retirement schemes continued even into the 1998-2000 period, when economic growth reached more than 8 % per year. The contradiction between low employment rate and one of the highest rates of GDP and employment growth in Europe over the recent period is explained by the flows of cross-border workers, who account for nearly 40 % of total employment.

The use of early retirement to absorb economic and social shocks continues to be supported by a strong, broad-based consensus between government, labour and management organisations within Luxembourg's model of tripartism. Although early retirements helped to address the crisis in the steel industry without increasing unemployment, this was done at a budgetary cost which was far from negligible. The sudden slowdown in economic activity since 2000 has led companies to freeze hiring and there have been many in-house plans to give the oldest workers individual incentives to retire on advantageous terms. The objective was to replace these retirees with younger, better-trained and more flexible resident or cross-border workers when business improves.

As a result, the employment rate has declined for workers between 50 and 64 years of age to 44 % in 2002. On the other hand, the overall employment rate for the 25-49 age group is slightly higher than the average for OECD countries.

1.3. Some steps in the right direction

Until now, the policy regarding the promotion of the employment of older workers has been to maintain the *status quo*. The Luxembourg authorities are nevertheless well aware of the fact that if no action is taken in this field there is a major risk of a widening gap with those European countries which have introduced new measures to promote the employment of older people. Luxembourg's influential tripartite body, the Economic and Social Council (CES), recently stated that "it is supportive of efforts aimed at increasing the employment rate of older people, which should ultimately lead to a lengthening of the average duration of working life, and which must go hand in hand with efforts by all players to increase the employability of older workers so as to maintain or improve the quality of work while respecting the state of workers' health" (CES, 2003b, p. 28).

Certain initiatives taken in recent years can be considered as steps in the right direction although these measures mostly apply to protraction of early retirement.

- More restrictive access to disability pensions since 1996 and, since the end of 2002, the requirement that persons with reduced capacity be redeployed in other jobs,
- introduction of a "premium" into the general pension scheme for persons with 38 years of contributions who continue working after the age of 55,
- measures to promote working until an older age in the civil service, and
- a workplace awareness-raising campaign against age-based discrimination.

1.4. A reluctance to act

The "wait-and-see" attitude of the government, employers and the trade unions in fact reflects a cautious stance on an issue that divides the social partners. On the one hand, employers see early retirement as a means of coping with short-term adjustment and controlling wage costs without too much opposition, and they propose maintaining early retirement schemes as exceptional measures that can be used in future situations of economic crisis. Trade unions, on the other hand, wish to expand these schemes so that they can cover all aspects of strenuous occupations experienced by workers as from the age of 55.

However, a policy of encouraging workers beyond the age of 50 to retire early is not in the interest of society, as early retirement schemes push up labour costs and impede the transfer of know-how. Production will increasingly rely on resident workers under 50 and cross-border workers, so undermining intergenerational solidarity. There is also a risk that expenditure on pensions may become unsustainable.

1.5. The need for a comprehensive reform package

Consequently a change is inevitable. A reform would require a policy of closer coordination between the relevant ministries (labour and employment, social affairs, education, finance) and an involvement of the social partners if restructuring is no longer to be managed by early retirement. A new social consensus will have to be established between the social partners and the government taking into account that social protection should no longer have the effect of undermining employment. Also vital are initiatives to improve working conditions, provide more training opportunities and make older people more employable.

To ensure that the reform makes headway, a few basic principles might provide some useful policy guidance. First, the government should clearly announce its intention to phase out passive early retirement measures and to use the resources for active measures to support the hiring of older workers or enable them to continue working. At the same time, steps should be taken to see what the Employment Administration (ADEM, *Administration de l'Emploi*) can do to help older workers to stay in or return to the labour market.

Consequently, the reform should focus on the following four areas:

- shifting away from the early retirement culture,
- reforming early-retirement schemes,
- encouraging employers to review their human resource management practices with regard to older workers, and
- continuing to promote employability among older members of the workforce.

1.5.1. Shifting away from the early retirement culture

To reverse the trend towards early retirement, all players should endorse a fundamental paradigm shift on employment schemes.

The following steps should therefore be taken without delay:

- *Launch a national campaign to change mentalities.* One priority would be to launch a nationwide campaign similar to Finland's; with the slogan "experience is a national asset". This campaign might focus on what older workers contribute to society.

- *Hold regular consultation meetings.* Consultation meetings could be a way of addressing, monitoring and coordinating effectively the cross cutting issue of jobs for older workers. The meetings should be attended by officials from the relevant institutions (employment, placement services, education, pensions, the economy and public finance).
- *Establish a database on older workers in order to analyse and target priority categories.* Any analysis of the situation of older workers in Luxembourg must overcome the problem that much data is not available by age.
- *Continue to conduct comprehensive studies on the ageing of the labour force.* Both the European peer review of Finland's national strategy towards older workers and the present Thematic Review are encouraging international initiatives that will enable Luxembourg to follow "best practices". The Labour Relations and Employment Observatory (ORPE) should be given additional financial resources to promote national evaluation studies.

1.5.2. Reforming early-retirement schemes

Although the reforms made to statutory pension schemes in the 1990s were steps in the right direction, the raising of pension levels decided in 2001 by the round table on pensions (*Rentendësch*) will not encourage workers to continue working beyond the minimum age of entitlement. This is 57 for workers with 40 years of actual service credit, and 60 for workers with 40 years of actual and attributed credit. As attributed years are granted very generously (up to nine years for higher education and ten years for the education of three children), many workers can retire at the age of 60. There is no deduction for early retirement at this age and the pension is the same as what would be paid at the age of 65.

A fundamental reform of the pension system must be initiated, as in Sweden (OECD, 2003b: see list of references on CD-ROM). Retirement decisions should be brought into line with longer life expectancy: the amount of pensions should be reduced in proportion to the number of years that retirement is taken before the legal age of 65, and the allowable number of years of attributed credit should be limited. Keeping individuals regularly informed of their pension entitlements would enable them to make informed choices.

In addition, for several decades the state has been using the Employment Fund to subsidise various pre-retirement schemes. The objective of reforms would be that companies taking advantage of a pre-retirement adjustment scheme should be required to bear a greater share of the costs resulting of early retirement benefits. Thus companies might also take active measures for training, reassignment or outplacement of workers in order to ensure effective planning based on the age profile of each company's workforce.

Moreover, the disability pension is currently used as a main scheme for withdrawing early from the labour market. In 1996, the medical criteria for granting a pension were enforced more stringently, and the number of new disability pensions granted was reduced by half. At the end of 2002, a scheme was established to help persons with reduced work capacity to re-enter the labour force. This type of reform appears to be potentially a promising method of reducing inactivity linked with disability pensions (OECD, 2003a, *Transforming Disability into Ability*).

In summary, the following measures should be given priority:

- *Carry out a basic reform of the general pension system.* This reform must be aimed at ensuring the system's long-term viability. The effective retirement age should be brought closer to the legal age of 65, and early retirement should be made more difficult and less financially attractive.
- *Limit the use of pre-retirement schemes as much as possible.* The government should make it more difficult for companies to use "*pre-retirement adjustment*" scheme (préretraite-ajustement) by requiring them to bear more of the occurring costs. The Employment Fund should be focused more on active measures to help older workers keep their job or find another one. A good example to follow in the processing of pre-retirement applications is that of the Joint Commission recently established to handle the redeployment of workers with reduced capacity.

2. Suggestions

2.1. Encouraging employers to review their human resource practices with regard to older workers

Firms must implement a new age-friendly employment policy that could help retain older members of the workforce, particularly more experienced workers. More emphasis should be placed on job interest, personal development and career prospects. For example, companies may be interested in taking advantage of older workers' ability to work independently by developing mentoring posts and audits and advisory duties suited to their skills, and by helping them to start a second career.

Encouraging employers to improve job quality and working conditions for all workers, irrespective of their age, is also important. Society as a whole will ultimately benefit by making jobs less arduous and better designed. Any improvement in working conditions will have an impact on the well-being at work. It will prevent the health of younger people from deteriorating prematurely and will help to keep ageing workers in employment.

Mutual learning based on good practices in companies and an exchange of views on the different strategies in OECD countries can help identify the most effective policies in this field.

Thus, corporate practices should be reviewed on the following basis:

- *Implement fully the European Directive on Age Discrimination, in consultation with the social partners.* The European Directive should fully ensure that the Criminal Code also prosecutes age discrimination in hiring, sanctioning or dismissing workers. However, the social partners should be consulted in order to ensure the legislation's effectiveness and minimise any additional costs for employers. The workplace awareness-raising campaign currently under way is a good start.
- *Challenge pay-practices based on age or length of service.* Social partners should be aware of the adverse effects that pay-scales linked only to age or length of service can have on the employment of older workers. Collective agreements should thus place more emphasis on skills and productivity.

- *Improve working conditions.* A tripartite consensus to create and finance a fund for promoting high-quality working conditions in general, and for older workers in particular, would be useful. For example, seniors should not be required to work night shifts.
- *Create and regularly update an Internet site devoted to good corporate practices.* The social partners, in cooperation with government, might disseminate good practices in companies via the Internet in order to promote the employment of older workers.

2.2. Continuing to promote the employability of older workers

Older workers are not a homogeneous group. Therefore it would be a mistake to rely on a single measure to help this group as a whole. In Luxembourg too few women continue to work after the age of 50. Thus specific measures could be adopted to help women who would like to resume working after raising a family. A reemployment measure such as that contained in the new Civil Service Regulations is an interesting step. Priority should also be given to part-time jobs and childcare services that will reconcile work and family life more easily. Workers should also been given the guarantee they will be reinstated in their former position after parental leave.

A gradual pre-retirement measure might also be studied and, in this regard, the reasons for the lack of success of the gradual pre-retirement scheme that has existed for a number of years in Luxembourg should be investigated.

The Public Employment Service, ADEM, should do more to help older unemployed workers to find jobs, making them a priority group and focusing on job search assistance. They should also promote the specific skills of older workers so as to counter employers' initial tendency to hire cross-border workers. Training counsellors to assist workers approaching retirement also appears to be a promising approach.

Expanding lifelong learning will be decisive for increasing labour force participation and retaining workers in employment longer. Vocational training has to become more an offensive and preventive means of promoting careers rather than to be seen as a defensive and palliative instrument against the risk of job loss or unemployment towards the end of one's working life. The social partners' recent agreement on improving individual access to continued training is thus a step in the right direction.

The following initiatives are recommended:

- *Make ADEM aware of older people's needs.* ADEM should focus more on offering jobs to seniors before turning towards cross-border workers. An evaluation of the hiring subsidy for older workers and long-term unemployed should be carried out.
- *Develop part-time work.* Opportunities for part-time work should be expanded and made more flexible in order to promote employment, especially for parents with young children and older workers. The measures taken in the public sector to help staff reconcile work and family life more easily are a step in the right direction.
- *Encourage greater participation in vocational training.* It will be crucial to increase participation by the entire workforce in high-quality training courses that will make all workers more employable throughout their working lives. On one hand, this will require more training provided by employers. On the other hand, if this training provides for recognised and valued skills at the labour market, participants should be willing to enrol in these courses and to shoulder part of the cost. Workers could be encouraged to participate financially through tax incentives.
- *Develop systems to recognise, certify and validate experience.* To develop the occupational competencies of older, relatively unskilled workers, it is vital to establish a recognition, certification and validation systems for the work-skills that they have gained, in many cases on the job.

The Netherlands

Lenneke Vaandrager, Elsa van der Maas

<table>
<tr><th>Field of promotion</th><th>Physical strain</th><th>Psyche / cognition</th><th>Mental / social competence</th><th>Professional competence</th></tr>
<tr><td>Action</td><td colspan="4"></td></tr>
<tr><td>Relief of physical strain / WHP actions</td><td colspan="2">Setting-based actions</td><td></td><td></td></tr>
<tr><td></td><td colspan="2">Behaviour-based actions *</td><td></td><td></td></tr>
<tr><td></td><td colspan="2">Integral health management</td><td></td><td></td></tr>
<tr><td></td><td colspan="2">Redundancy protection - fewer repetitive tasks</td><td></td><td></td></tr>
<tr><td></td><td colspan="2">Task reduction</td><td></td><td></td></tr>
<tr><td></td><td>Micro-breaks</td><td></td><td></td><td></td></tr>
<tr><td></td><td colspan="3">Work ability index</td><td></td></tr>
<tr><td>Age-related working hours</td><td colspan="2">Reduction of working hours</td><td></td><td></td></tr>
<tr><td></td><td colspan="2">Exemption from shift working</td><td></td><td></td></tr>
<tr><td></td><td colspan="2">Exemption from working overtime</td><td></td><td></td></tr>
<tr><td></td><td colspan="2">Additional days off (according to labour agreements)</td><td></td><td></td></tr>
<tr><td></td><td colspan="2">Lifetime working schemes</td><td></td><td></td></tr>
<tr><td></td><td colspan="2">Part-time employment / retirement</td><td></td><td></td></tr>
<tr><td></td><td colspan="4">Age proof jobs (balance between decreasing and increasing abilities during one's professional life)</td></tr>
<tr><td>Qualification</td><td></td><td colspan="3">Knowledge management / transfer
("Young Head on Old Shoulders")</td></tr>
<tr><td></td><td></td><td colspan="3">Aged become "On-the-job-trainers"</td></tr>
</table>

<table>
<tr><th>Field of promotion</th><th>Physical strain</th><th>Psyche / cognition</th><th>Mental / social competence</th><th>Professional competence</th></tr>
<tr><td></td><td></td><td colspan="3">Lifelong learning</td></tr>
<tr><td></td><td colspan="4">Structural help for seniors to start their own enterprises</td></tr>
<tr><td></td><td colspan="4">Support of staff with individual development</td></tr>
<tr><td>Communication</td><td></td><td colspan="3">Raise management competence</td></tr>
<tr><td></td><td colspan="4">Age diversity management (career, job content, working environment)</td></tr>
<tr><td></td><td colspan="4">Age mirror, age profiling (estimation on future age composition within a company)</td></tr>
<tr><td></td><td colspan="4">Age awareness in company's policy</td></tr>
<tr><td></td><td colspan="4">Avoiding age discrimination in job application or in-house applications</td></tr>
<tr><td></td><td colspan="4">Conscious absenteeism policy</td></tr>
<tr><td></td><td colspan="4">Correction of prejudices concerning aged</td></tr>
</table>

* *Exercise, nutrition, consumption of alcohol and nicotine, relaxation*

Fig. 14: Summary of actions - The Netherlands

1. Political basis

Measures

Financial measures taken by the government to make a longer working life more attractive and to discourage early retirement are currently subject to considerable change.

The measures are also aimed at encouraging employers to keep or hire older employees. (http://home.szw.nl/index/dsp_index.cfm, 8.9.2004)

Financial incentives

- *Early Retirement (VUT) and pre-pension schemes:* from January 1, 2006, employees are no longer obliged to contribute to the pre-pension funds. In time, the cabinet will no longer give fiscal support to the pre-pension schemes. This scheme will be replaced by the course-of-life scheme.
- *WW (Unemployment Benefit):* from January 1, 2005, the dismissal allowance - with the exception of schooling costs - will be deducted from the Unemployment Benefit (WW-benefit).
- *Abolition of the continued unemployment benefit (WW):* from January 1, 2004, the continued unemployment benefit WW has been abolished for people who have become unemployed on or after August 11, 2003. Older employees were entitled to continued unemployment benefit for 3.5 years at most. The abolition of the continued unemployment benefit restricts the exceptional position of employees who are 57.5 years and older when they become unemployed, and encourages the resumption of work.
- *Raising the minimum age for the IOAW[5] from 50 to 55 years of age:* the cabinet intends a preventive effect for employees who are threatened with dismissal. An employee at the age of

[5] The IOAW is a minimum level financial provision for elderly unemployed workers and people with an occupational disability which they are entitled to once they are no longer eligible for unemployment benefits.

50-55 years will not consent to dismissal so easily knowing that, after the WW (Unemployment Benefit) period, he first has to break into his own reserves before he can apply for social security payment. But also during the WW (Unemployment Benefit) period people affected will go looking for jobs more actively in order to prevent welfare.

- *The obligation to apply for jobs for 57.5 year-olds who are on WW (Unemployment Benefit):* from January 1, 2004, employees who become unemployed at the age of 57.5 years or more have the same obligations (e.g. the obligation to apply for jobs) to seek and accept jobs as any other unemployed person.
- *The obligation to apply for jobs for 57.5 year-olds in the WWB (Work and Social security Act):* from January 1, 2004, people on social security who are 57.5 years old or older have to apply for jobs. This was reintroduced with the Work and Social Security Act.
- *Legal right to a "division-regulation":* acquired pension rights must not be lost if employees want to take a step back in their career. The result of this regulation is the division of times of employment into several periods. The right to a division-regulation will be included in the new pension law that is currently being prepared. The aim is to submit the new pension law to the Lower Chamber in 2005.
- *A specific labour credit for older people:* it has been made more attractive for older people to keep working because of the introduction in 2002 of a specific labour credit for older people which becomes higher with age. The monthly fiscal benefit for employees from 57 up to 64 years amounts to € 18.90 at 57 and increases to € 56.80 at 64 years.
- *Daily wage guarantee WW:* on the basis of the daily wage guarantee scheme, a released employee who resumes lower paid work within 12 months gets an allowance based on the old, higher daily wage if unemployed later. For employees who are 57.5 years old and older, the period of the guarantee extends until their 65th year. The age limit of 57.5 years will further be lowered to 55 years. This scheme reduces the risk

of lower unemployment benefit when accepting lower paid work and thereby stimulates the fast resumption of work. This measure has come into force on January 1, 2005.
- *Reform of the WAO (Occupational Disability Insurance Act):* no specific measures on the subject of unemployment benefit conditions for older employees. A number of points have been adjusted. Only the working, partially disabled are entitled to a wage supplementation scheme. Especially for older employees this will be an additional impulse to keep working longer.
- *Premium exemption for older workers:* came into force on January 1, 2004, and gives employers an exemption from the WAO (Occupational Disability Insurance Act) basic premium for employees who are 50 years or older when they take up employment. Employers also get a premium exemption for their employees of 55 years or older.

Concerning industrial law, the government has not given much thought (yet) about hiring over-65s or keeping them employed. Legal insecurity in this cause prevails and many employers see too many risks in connection with the employment of workers of 65 years and older: in case of ill health, the employer is obliged to continue payments. This is considered very expensive, especially when it entails hiring new personnel. As a result almost all employees still working at the age of 65 and over are working on the basis of temporary contracts; either through their employer, or through a temp-agency. (www.leeftijd.nl)

2. National programmes / projects

The cabinet has brought some national programmes into being to stimulate a longer working career for elderly. Examples are the Taskforce Older People and Labour, which is now discontinued, and the accompanying Cum L'Oude award, the promotion scheme for age-conscious policy and the EQUAL-programme. These are mentioned below.

2.1. The Taskforce Older People and Labour

The Taskforce Older People and Labour (TOA), which is now discontinued, formulated recommendations in the period 2001-2003, to remove obstacles to a greater participation in the employment market for older people. It was about the realisation of age-conscious policy, the employability of older people, financial incentives and the implementation of the recommendations. These have been laid down with social partners, authorities, implementing institutions and individual citizens. (www.ouderenenarbeid.nl)

The Taskforce Older People and Employment's final report delivers a lot of recommendations for keeping older workforce longer and more healthy in employment. Amongst these are:

- Integral health management: with shifting emphasis more on prevention annual cost for absenteeism and disability benefits will decrease and personal well-being will be increased (see section 3.3.1. TNO Arbeid).
- Redundancy protection could be carried out through better cross-sector mobility of staff.
- Fewer repetitive occupational tasks will contribute to continued employability of older workers.
- Part-time employment/retirement is stressed to be essential for better health in an advanced age.
- Knowledge management/transfer is suggested according to the example of Deutsche Bank's "Know-How Teams"; Taskforce calls this recommendation "Young Heads on Old Shoulders" by adding that people who are better educated are more productive.
- Therefore Lifelong Learning is another issue that would raise older workers' employability.
- Age awareness in company's policy and therefore also avoiding age discrimination in recruitment schemes is also stressed as crucial for employees' as well as employer's benefit.

(http://www.ouderenenarbeid.nl/artman/uploads/recommendationsinstrumentseng.pdf)

2.2. Cum l'Oude Award

The Cum l'Oude award (http://www.cumloude.nl/) was created by the Taskforce Older People, set up by the Minister for Social Services and Employment in order to trace and reward age-friendly policies in organisations. The winner of the Cum L'Oude Award of 2003 was the Milieudienst Groningen (see section 4.).

2.3. Encouragement scheme for an age-conscious policy

There are still not very many companies that actively pursue an age-conscious policy. Many employers expect that the age structure in companies will remain the same in the future.

Therefore a stimulation scheme of the Ministry of Social Affairs and Employment has been designed to remove obstacles for the longer employment of older people. Obstacles could be prejudices and negative stereotypes, design of the workplace or content of the job, low career opportunities and long-term pressure on employees. The Taskforce Older People and Labour has recommended a number of instruments (for example age mirror, age-proof jobs, talent plus, CAO [Collective Labour Agreement] recommendations for the sustained deployment of people of all ages) that form a good base for future policy on age awareness. (www.agentschap.szw.nl/, 24.11.2004)

The scheme has come into force on December 1, 2004, and will run until 2007. It will especially concentrate on the topics conceptualisation, realisation and agenda-setting. The aim is to make sure that employers make optimal use of the funds made available for the scheme to promote an age-conscious policy. Available in total: € 21 million, up to a maximum of € 50,000 per application.

Within the framework of the scheme, pilot projects will also be started on inter-sector mobility in several regions in the Netherlands.

2.4. EQUAL Programme

Within the framework of this European programme, projects have been funded for developing new instruments and procedures in order to promote labour participation of older people (www.europa.eu.int). In project proposals, a change in thinking has been favoured about older people, employers and trade unions, intermediaries for the labour participation of older people.

So far a total of 98 projects have been honoured in the Netherlands. The project "Verbreding Werkwijzer" (Senior Professionals Wiser at Work) could serve as an example here. The organisation PSW Arbeidsmarktadvies (PSW Labour Market Advice) in Breda has developed the concept "WerkWijzer" by which attention is drawn to measures for keeping older people at work or getting them to work again. Supported by the European Commission (EQUAL), the Taskforce Older People and contributions from that region, this concept has been used in seven other regions. Older employees throughout the Netherlands and job-seekers as well as employers now can get information and advice on keeping over-45ers on the labour market and on how over-45ers can re-enter the labour market. (www.wwijzer.nl)

3. Players

3.1. NGOs / interest group representatives

Bureaus and knowledge centres are increasingly offering services that are aimed at the promotion of the labour participation of older people.

3.1.1. Service point Labour Market SME (Small and Medium-sized Enterprises)

The Service point Labour Market SME is a collaboration between the National Centre for Work and Income (CWI), MKB Nederland and the Ministry of Social Affairs and Employment. In a series of presentations, articles in branch magazines, personal contacts and a special matching project for the fashion retail trade (www.servicepunktmkb.nl/ouderen) the service point provides information on the ageing of the labour market for employees of SMEs.

3.1.2. The LBL, Expert Centre Age and Society

The LBL, Expert Centre Age and Society, is an independent expert centre that, by means of acquiring and diffusing knowledge on the course of life, age and age limits, contributes to a multiform society in which people can organise their course of life to their own choice and in which unjustified age discrimination does not exist. By order of the Taskforce Older People and Labour, the LBL, Expert Centre Age and Society, has listed the possibilities for CAO (Collective Labour Agreements) agreements that contribute to the promotion of an activating personnel policy for all ages.

In the period 2004-2005, the LBL is carrying out the project "Age and Labour: towards a sustained deployment of people of all ages". The aim of this project is to promote the sustainable deployment of people of all ages, with special attention to older people. By means of this project an important contribution is made to the implementation of the Equal Treatment Act on the basis of age in employment. The LBL plays an important role in the implementation of this Act.

The report will contain a large number of recommendations social partners can work with in the CAO-consultation. The recommendations fit in with recognisable themes in the consultation on conditions of employment, such as employability, arbo policies (occupational health and safety) and course of life.

Examples are task reduction, reduction of working hours and exemption from working in shifts or working overtime. Promotion of age diversity management and the introduction of a specific employability policy are addressed in the report; additionally, improvements in the working conditions and health in the company and introduction of course-of-life schemes are recommended. From a certain age on (different for various Agreements) a right to extra paid vacation is granted. As a good alternative for this one-sided approach LBL stresses the model for sustainable taxability. (www.leeftijd.nl; 15.11.04)

3.1.3. Opportunity in Business & the National Network Diversity Management

Opportunity in Business is a national network of companies and organisations that are working on a balanced composition of their personnel. The national network Diversity Management (DIV) is part of this network. The

DIV will be actively advising employers on age-conscious personnel policy. (www.opportunity.nl)

3.1.4. National Centre for Work and Income (CWI)

The National Centre for Work and Income (CWI) has developed a special information module for older people by order of the Ministry of Social Affairs and Employment. This module is aimed at older employees and the employers who want to hire them. (www.werk.nl)

3.1.5. UWV

The UWV basically does not operate a specific target group policy, but tailor-made solutions. Older people can get intensive help concerning reintegration within the framework of this tailor-made solution approach. In addition it is ensured that older people who are going to follow a reintegration programme will enter a reintegration institution that is especially aimed at older people (Eindrapportage Taskforce ouderen en arbeid, 2003).

3.1.6. Federation Dutch Trade Unions (FNV)

Comprising fourteen unions jointly representing the interests of over 1.2 million members, the FNV is by far the largest trade union confederation in the Netherlands. By order of the FNV, the University of Utrecht conducted the study "Carrying on working with policy" (Leisink, 2004). One of the findings of this survey is that an older employee working under a competent manager feels less need to retire early. In addition, by order of the FNV, a scan for policies in human resource management was developed. By means of this instrument companies can test and optimise their policies for older people. At the end of 2004 the scan will be ready for use. (www.fnv.nl/40+, www.40plusloonwijzer.nl, 14.11.04)

3.1.7. PSW Arbeidsmartktadvies (PSW Labour Market Advice)

PSW Arbeidsmarktadvies (www.psw.nl) aims at getting people who are at risk on the labour market back to work and keeping them in work. PSW Arbeidsmarktadvies is not an implementing institution but takes new initiatives and provides information, support and advice. This bureau developed a project on the deployment of older people as practical instructors: experienced professionals teach freshmen the tricks of the trade. Further the PSW has developed the concept WerkWijzer, regional support offices for employees over 45 years old (see EQUAL Programme).

3.1.8. The Bureau for Demography and Innovation (Demin)

Demin aims at promoting the labour participation of older people and emphasises the knowledge and expertise that older workers bring. Demin combines expertise and offers access to networks; it supports and develops innovative pilots and projects, especially but not exclusively in the area of demographic changes. To this end Demin cooperates with partners in Europe and the U.S. (www.demin.biz)

3.1.9. Network "Work Ability Index"

The Network "Work Ability Index" (in establishment) promotes the deployment of the Work Ability Index in the Netherlands within the frameworks of health policy (keeping people healthy and keeping them able to work longer). This is an instrument to measure the (future) capability of employees. Within this network, work will be done on the organisation of the aforementioned information, organising meetings and the support and organisation of training and the mutual exchange of users. The Finnish developer of the WAI is willing to give the copyright to the network under the condition of quality control (Notitie Oprichting Netwerk Work Ability Index, 2004).

3.1.10. Netherlands Institute for Health Promotion and Disease Prevention (NIGZ)

The NIGZ (Netherlands Institute for Health Promotion and Disease Prevention) develops programmes in support of healthy behaviour and healthy environments. The NIGZ especially assist local authorities, local health promoting institutions and companies in developing, implementing and assessing health policies.

The work is inspired by the Ottawa Charter for Health Promotion, in which health promotion has been described as "the process of enabling people to increase control over, and to improve, their health".

The Dutch Centre for Workplace Health Promotion has become a division of the NIGZ, as NIGZ Work & Health. In close European cooperation, as being the Dutch contact office of the European Network for Workplace Health Promotion, NIGZ Work & Health will continue its projects and programmes for healthy lifestyles and healthy working environments.

NIGZ Work and Health promotes WHP through educational programmes, training and information; and guides WHP policies at the workplace level. These programmes are mostly aimed at lifestyle determinants like smoking, nutrition, exercise, alcohol and pure air.

3.2. Private / commercial service enterprises

More and more commercial bureaus will be occupied with the subject of age policy. However, there are too many to describe and therefore the following selection has to serve the purpose.

3.2.1. GOC knowledge centre

GOC is the knowledge centre for education, the labour market and training & advice in the graphics-media branch. The number of older workers in the graphics industry is rising steadily. In order to anticipate this, the GOC knowledge centre is working on awareness-raising. They are engaged in developing various management instruments and hold meetings for works councils. (http://www.goc.nl/ and http://www.arbografimedia.nl/)

Project Age Unlimited:

GOC knowledge centre offers people in the WAO and the WW (in the graphics-media branch) counselling and training to help them get back to work again. The project motivates employers and employees to work together at activities.

3.2.2. Bureau Ageproof

AgeProof is a bureau that is engaged with the ageing of personnel in organisations and its expertise concerns sustained employability policy. AgeProofing stands for the methodical adjustment of functions, adjusting work to a better balance of life on and off the job. It is a method to improve the age stability of functions. For this project 40 functions have been analysed on age stability up to now. (www.ageproof.nl)

3.2.3. Temp-agency for Seniors "Outstanding"

The temp-agency "Outstanding" brings employers' need of a good telephonist/receptionist together with enthusiastic and suitable older job-seekers. Brief training and coaching are provided before and after people start working. (www.outstanding.nl)

3.2.4. Seniorstart Nederland

In cooperation with the foundation Wise, MKB Nederland has developed a regional office for elderly starting their own enterprise. The main goal is exchanging experiences, effective support for seniors in starting their own company and developing regional knowledge networks. A network of colleagues is the perfect background to help over-45ers with starting their own company. In a number of regions networks have already been formed or are in the course of formation. (www.kenniscentrumouderen.amsterdam.nl/ and www.seniorstart.org/)

3.3. Research organisations

A lot of research has been done in the area of age policy and what kind of measures could be taken so that older people can carry on working healthily and happily. Below a number of important research bureaus and the research they have done are described.

3.3.1. TNO Arbeid (TNO Work & Employment) / STECR

TNO Arbeid is engaged in knowledge development, research, advice and implementation of solutions for problems at work. A lot of research concerns older people and older people at work as well. For example, in May 2004, the National Survey on Working Conditions was conducted. The theme "Carrying on working until the 65th year of life" has also been taken onto the agenda. It became clear that health is the most important prerequisite to carry on working longer. (www.arbeid.tno.nl; 14.11.04)

In addition TNO Arbeid has recently (2004) published the report "De mythe doorbroken. Gezondheid en inzetbaarheid oudere werknemers" ("The myth break through. Health and availability (usability) of older employees"). By order of the Taskforce Older People and Labour "TNO Arbeid" listed what employees of a higher age need to be able to work vitally, healthily and happily (Nauta et al., 2004).

At STECR (www.stecr.nl/ "Platform Reïntegratie" - Platform Reintegration) professionals can share their knowledge and experiences around reintegration. It is an initiative of the Branch Organisation Arbo-services (BOA), supported by the Ministry of Social Affairs and Employment, TNO Arbeid and Nationale Nederlanden. In June 2004, STECR published the study report "The older employee. Dealing with ageing in the organisation". Some conclusions from this report are that there is the urgent issue of the ageing of the labour force and that this problem will increase further in the future. It was stated that the image of older people at work is unnecessarily negative for employers and younger employees. It is essential that branch organisations, employers and employees take action on this issue (Hidding et al., 2004).

3.3.2. SEO (Foundation for Economic Research, www.seo.nl/)

By order of the Regional Platform Labour Market Policy of Southern North Holland, the research institution SEO made an inventory of the basics of age policy in the provincial labour market. From this report it appears that in the next twenty years, as one result of ageing, a significant deficit of experienced employees will arise. Therefore older employees will become a necessary source for the labour market. Keeping older people at work becomes more effective when the relationship between the costs and productivity of older employees is improved and the reasons for early retirement are suppressed. This means, on the one hand, a saving in (expensive) early retirement procedures and, on the other hand, an investment in education and career development (Heyma, et al., 2003).

3.3.3. Scholar

The Taskforce Older People and Labour asked the University of Amsterdam to take stock of published scientific researches on the problem of older people and employment and to analyse the usefulness of these publications. Resulting is the report "Winst komt met jaren" (Age comes with gains) which lists conclusions and recommendations on the topic. "Scholar" is an institute for training, labour market and economic development of the University of Amsterdam. The researchers of the institute plead for more targeted training of older employees to increase their productivity (Eindrapportage Taskforce Ouderen en Arbeid, 2003).

3.3.3.1. University of Utrecht

By order of the FNV (Dutch Trades Union Congress) the research entitled "Carrying on working with policy" was carried out (2004, see FNV under section 3.1.6.).

3.3.3.2. Tangram and Signs of the Time

The workplace professionals have examined emotions concerning early retirement and carrying on working beyond that age. The ageing and dejuvenation in society are forcing more people to carry on working till, and even beyond, their 66th year. In the survey carried out by order of the Taskforce Older People and Labour the perception of getting older and nevertheless carrying on working is mapped. The aim of this research was to find out how the current and future generations of older people can be persuaded to work longer.

The report highlights that payment is not always the primary reason to work. Respect and appreciation for the commitment which older employees show and the performance they accomplish, linked to more flexibility and freedom in the division of work, appear to be the most effective means to motivate employees to carry on working longer. (www.tangram.nl/)

3.3.3.3. Coronel Institute

This institute carries out research on factors in the working situation that contribute to the continuation of physiological and psychological reactivity after work ("spill-over"). Part of the research and development activities is aimed at norms for workplace health promotion. A special area of attention within this theme is "Ageing and Work".

By order of the SOVAM, the sector fund for ambulance care, research has been conducted within the ambulance sector, in order to give suggestions on new policies for older staff. As existing policies are aimed at collective early retirement, new scientific research demonstrates that there cannot be a certain collective age at which working on ambulances becomes too hard, either physically or mentally. On the other hand, it seems obvious that for some employees this kind of work can become too strenuous long before the current age of retirement of 55 years. In order to make sure that employees of any age keep working in a good state of health an individual approach is essential. The employers suggest to the unions to examine employees periodically and transfer them in time to a less strenuous job. Thus the Coronel Institute developed specific norms for periodic labour health studies for older employees in the building industry and norms for adjustment of working time of older employees. (www.amc.nl/ and www.vng.nl/ 30.8.2004)

3.3.3.4. Bureau Astri

Astri is a private and independent bureau for policy research and advice in the area of social insurance, labour and health. Astri works for private, social and insurance bodies, national authorities, sector organisations in business, social partners and international organisations and also carries out research in the area of age-conscious policy. (www.astri.nl/)

4. Projects

Quite a few organisations already envision the benefits of keeping older employees in employment. Siemens won the LABOR Award in 2002. This price was later turned into the Cum L'Oude award, which has been described above. The Milieudienst Groningen won this award in 2003. The other two projects described here are the green grey policy and policies for older people in labour organisations.

4.1. Siemens (www.siemens.nl/)

Siemens is a multinational and is active in almost all areas of electro-technology and electronics in the Netherlands. In 2003, it employed a staff of 3,094.

Siemens has structural attention for the safety, health and well-being of its employees for 20 years now. The background is that the more an employee is mentally and physically fit, the more creative and resilient he will be and so will meet new challenges much better.

Workplace health promotion is an integrated part of Siemens' business activities. Important elements are the intensive support of employees in their development and the promotion of flow-through. Siemens is pursuing a conscious absenteeism policy; absenteeism support is not given to an external occupational safety and health service but kept an in-house agenda. It is regularly evaluated by means of surveys of the appreciation of employees and by means of the assessment of executives by employees.

At the beginning of 2003, Siemens Nederland was certified as a "Model of Good Practice" by the Dutch Centre for Workplace Health Promotion (now the NIGZ - Work & Health) for their WHP-policy.

In addition, Siemens received the LABOR Award for age-conscious personnel policy (renamed in Cum L'Oude Award) in 2002. Siemens received this award because it has not implemented a separate policy for older staff, as this differentiation stigmatises the older members of the workforce. (Presbericht: Siemens Nederland opnieuw gecertificeerd tot Europees "Model of Good Practice" voor gezondheidsbeleid - Press release: Siemens Holland certified again for European "Model of Good Practice" for health policy)

4.2. Milieudienst (Environmental Service) Groningen

The Milieudienst Groningen collects waste in the city of Groningen. Within this service a lot of attention is given to the development and training of employees, change of tasks and a broad employability. For example, employees will only obtain a permanent appointment if they have successfully completed a number of training sessions. Depending on age, an employee either does or no longer carries out physically challenging work (till the age of 30 employees can be fully deployed in the loading of dustbin bags, employees from 30 till 40 years of age only for 50 % of working hours and above the age of 40 they will have other tasks). Employees who can no longer work in the field are deployed as coaches for younger colleagues (Nauta et al., 2004).

4.3. Green Grey Policy: Optimal Return of Young and Old

Bureau Ageproof has developed a five-step plan for green-grey policy. This plan should indicate how things can be improved within a certain organisation so that both younger and older employees can be deployed optimally.

The following example serves as an illustration of this approach.

In a utility company in the North of the Netherlands over 60 % of the employees were older than 45 years. The majority of them had been in employment for over 20 years. More and more older employees went on (early) retirement. Because of the scarcity on the labour market, taking on sufficient new staff became a problem. In the early nineties the demand for assistant mechanics, who mainly carry out heavy physical work, decreased. At the same time the demand increased for skilled, independently working mechanics who were able to supervise. In order to prevent the loss of assistant mechanics and to fulfil the demand for mechanics, the company started up a project in which the assistant mechanics (with an average age of 45 years) were retrained or were given further training to be a mechanic.

The most important benefits from this project were:

- Making use of the skills of older employees. As a result their motivation increased, the physical strain decreased, absenteeism went down, productivity went up and the service and delivery performance improved.
- Achieving equality of rights for assistant mechanics who were already doing mechanics' work, but were not rewarded for it as such.
- A saving in costs for the recruitment, selection, settlement, and training of new personnel.
- The balance of costs and benefits in this project turned out to be positive.

(http://www.ageproof.nl/)

4.4. Research: Policies for Older People Organisations

By order of the FNV (Federation Dutch Trade Union), researchers from the University of Utrecht carried out a study concerning the characteristics of policies for older people in organisations. Emphasis is given to the question which measures are realised most in the practice of labour organisations.

One company that has taken part in this research is quite a large company in the painting branch. It employs 109 people, 95 of which are painters.

The reason for participating in this research is the management's awareness of the fact that 25 % of staff is already older than 50 years. The increased attention to older workforce accrues from the company's costs related to the WAO (Occupational Disability Insurance Act) and from a greater independence of the older people themselves.

Within this company great importance to training is attached; 100 employees took part in some kind of training in 2002.

The work is divided in such a way that older staff do not have to climb too much any more and, if possible, do not have to work outside in the rain or cold. The construction of scaffolds has been contracted out and heavy work is avoided where possible. Project managers see to it that safety measures are taken seriously.

In addition the director emphasises there is no policy aimed at persons leaving at the VUT[6]-age, because older colleagues can instruct younger ones a lot, both in painting and related physical work and in the contact with clients. It is important that regulations for older workers are included in the CAO (Collective Labour Agreement), which make it possible to keep older employees working longer. Therefore the company sees to it that employees make use of those schemes, like additional days off. There is hardly any turnover of labour with this company; so it is possible to tie the personnel to this company permanently.

One factor hindering its policy is that there are few possibilities for function differentiation. Executives and employees do not think that working longer than the early retirement age in the current CAO is desirable, because of the health interests of the employees and the fact that most of the employees started working at a young age (Leisink et al., 2003).

[6] VUT stands for early retirement.

Norway

Odd Bjørnstad

<table>
<tr><th>Field of promotion</th><th>Physical strain</th><th>Psyche / cognition</th><th>Mental / social competence</th><th>Professional competence</th></tr>
<tr><td>Action</td><td colspan="4"></td></tr>
<tr><td>Relief of physical strain / WHP actions</td><td colspan="2">Setting-based measures</td><td></td><td></td></tr>
<tr><td></td><td colspan="2">Behaviour-based measures *</td><td></td><td></td></tr>
<tr><td></td><td colspan="4">"Inclusive Workplaces"
changing skills, attitude, culture to adapt to age and disabilities (management and employees)</td></tr>
<tr><td></td><td colspan="3">Internal control: systematic health, safety and environmental programmes</td><td></td></tr>
<tr><td></td><td colspan="4">Age-related human resource management and work environment</td></tr>
<tr><td></td><td colspan="4">Creation of extra senior sections</td></tr>
<tr><td></td><td colspan="3">One hour physical training exercise per week when over 60 years old</td><td></td></tr>
<tr><td>Age-related working hours</td><td colspan="2">More flexible retirement regulations</td><td></td><td></td></tr>
<tr><td></td><td colspan="3">No overtime work for elders</td><td></td></tr>
<tr><td></td><td colspan="3">Three extra days off when over 60 years old</td><td></td></tr>
<tr><td></td><td colspan="3">Shorter working days when over 64 years old</td><td></td></tr>
<tr><td></td><td colspan="4">Home office work as an option</td></tr>
<tr><td>Qualification</td><td colspan="4">Senior training - personal and professional</td></tr>
<tr><td></td><td colspan="4">Senior career planning</td></tr>
<tr><td></td><td colspan="4">Privilege for older workers to gain formal qualification before younger ones - due to tutorship</td></tr>
<tr><td></td><td colspan="4">Senior advicers</td></tr>
</table>

<table>
<tr><th>Field of promotion</th><th>Physical strain</th><th>Psyche / cognition</th><th>Mental / social competence</th><th>Professional competence</th></tr>
<tr><td>Communication</td><td colspan="4">Age equality company policy</td></tr>
<tr><td></td><td colspan="4">Establishing a senior committee for planning altered job arrangements and retirement forms</td></tr>
<tr><td></td><td colspan="3">Intranet page presenting senior policy information</td><td></td></tr>
<tr><td></td><td colspan="3">Personal interviews dealing with senior policy topics</td><td></td></tr>
<tr><td></td><td colspan="4">Providing union representatives with training in senior work environments</td></tr>
<tr><td></td><td></td><td colspan="3">Age-awareness / information campaigns</td></tr>
<tr><td></td><td></td><td colspan="3">Developing information materials (handbooks, magazines etc.)</td></tr>
<tr><td></td><td></td><td colspan="3">Conferences on problems of older workers</td></tr>
<tr><td></td><td></td><td colspan="3">Special fund for age-related studies</td></tr>
</table>

** Exercise, nutrition, consumption of alcohol and nicotine, relaxation*

Fig. 15: Summary of actions - Norway

1. Political basis

1.1. Tripartite agreement on a more inclusive workplace

The Tripartite Agreement on a "More Inclusive Workplace" was signed by the social partners and authorities in Norway in October 2001. The general objectives were:

- to reduce sickness absence,
- to provide employment to a far greater number of employees whose functional capacity is impaired than is the case today, and
- to raise the real retirement age (i.e. the average age of retirement from working life).

An "Inclusive Workplace" is a workplace which has room for everyone who wants to and is able to work. There must be room for people with temporary or permanent disabilities as well as for older employees. The responsibility for promoting an inclusive work environment must be rooted in the workplace.

This means organising and facilitating the work in a way which enables as many employees as possible to function in their jobs and cope with their work tasks. It also means focusing specifically on skills, attitudes and culture. Managers have a special responsibility in this context, but also individual employees have to do their part and utilise their capacity for work to the best of their ability. By helping each other and working together, a good work environment can be created. Therefore everyone has to make their own needs known and by exploiting the possibilities and measures available at the workplace their needs should be satisfied to the greatest possible extent.

The employers and the union representatives/employees' representatives will jointly set specific objectives for the enterprises under each of the general objectives.

Efforts to achieve a more inclusive workplace are part of the enterprise's systematic health, safety and environment programme (internal control).

At present 57 % of the workforce is working in enterprises which have joined the agreement on a more inclusive workplace.

The sick leave rate for these enterprises has decreased.
But the third objective, to raise the real retirement age, has not been reached yet. No figures show an increase in the retirement age.

2. National programmes / projects

2.1. The Centre for Senior Policy

Since 1969, the Centre for Senior Policy (CSP) has been engaged in running courses preparing workers for retirement. Now the efforts are directed towards a wider personnel policy area, including groups from age 45 and over, called "seniors".

The present purpose of CSP is to make individuals, companies and politicians aware of the benefits of accommodating workers over the age of 45, as they are an increasing proportion of the workforce.

Through promoting research, awareness campaigns and by forging links between labour unions, employer associations and politicians, CSP encourages a wide range of activities whose aim it is to reverse the growing trend towards early retirement.

Establishing "alliances" has been of the greatest importance. By stimulating activities, making people aware of personal and professional development, by encouraging training of seniors and senior career planning, they hope to reduce seniors' premature departure from the workforce, and to increase their ability to cope with change. The aim is to build up an awareness of the potential of the senior workforce in general personnel policy in Norway.

In practice, the CSP has been a central partner and coordinator for public and private enterprises. Valuable experience and competency have been gained through projects in the last 10 years.

2.2. National Initiative for Senior Workers in Norway

National Initiative for Senior Workers is part of the strategy aimed at the top management of all the major unions and employers' associations and relevant government agencies. The government will give annual financial support to this national plan for the years 2001-2005.

In order to prevent the exclusion of older workers before retirement age the government wanted in this way to encourage employers to provide a better working environment for older workers and to introduce age-related HR management.

In brief, the plan consists of the following elements which the organisations have committed themselves to:

- using their branches actively in spreading information, appropriate models, practical experience and research results in the area of senior personnel policy,
- arranging conferences and training for respective target groups, and
- providing union representatives with training in senior work environments.

In addition there will be activities in a national plan:

- information campaigns,
- organisational development projects,
- models of good practice,
- networks, and
- development of handbooks and other materials.

The Centre for Senior Policy is responsible for coordinating the National Initiative for Senior Workers.

2.3. The National Council for Senior Citizens

The National Council for Senior citizens is an advisory body for public authorities and national institutions, and opens up discussions on a free and independent basis on issues concerning the living conditions of senior citizens and their possibilities for taking part in working life and society as a whole. In particular the Council will concentrate on aspects of care for elders and policy for senior citizens that affect persons with special needs for nursing and care. In this context senior citizen means persons approximately 50 years old.

The Council will:
- afford ground for debate between the members of the Council and representatives for public authorities and national institutions on issues concerning senior citizens' situation in society,
- generate and express opinions on important issues concerning senior citizens,
- obtain information about needs, problems and possible solutions at the local, regional and central level, enabling it to take initiative and give advice to public authorities and national institutions, and
- provide information to the public in general.

The Council is administratively subordinated to the Ministry of Social Affairs, and has its own secretary as provided by the Ministry.

3. Players

3.1. NGOs / interest group representatives

3.1.1. Senior Policy Network

The Network is a forum for learning and exchanging experience within the field of seniors in working life. It should give inspiration and motivation for further engagement for the members to work within their own organisations.

Persons involved in the Network are representatives from
- the National Insurance Service,
- enterprises active working with senior policy,
- Centre for Senior Policy, and
- private consultants.

In Norwegian: Seniorpolitisk nettverk (www.idebanken.org/viken2.asp or http://www.idebanken.org/default.asp?show=art&artID=1188)

3.1.2. Norwegian Pensioners Association (NPA)

NPA is the largest association of pensioners in Norway, having over 150,000 members. They run more than one thousand local clubs, spread all over the country and in all municipalities, as well as regional offices in each of Norway's 19 counties. NPA was founded in 1952 and is politically neutral. The association has an exclusive right to negotiate directly with the government on behalf of the pensioners in economical, social and cultural matters. NPA considers itself an active participant in the national, regional and local politics of the elderly. The idea of contributing to welfare of society is a very important idea in the Norwegian Pensioners Association. Having its focus on life in retirement NPA doesn't work on questions regarding ageing workforce and workplaces.

In Norwegian: Pensjonistforbundet (www.pensjonistforbundet.no).

3.1.3. The Norwegian Senior Citizen Association

The Norwegian Senior Citizen Association is a special interest organisation which wants to influence the authorities and national politicians to make decisions appropriate for seniors in working life.

They are working for a more flexible retirement pension and jobs for both young people and seniors. A society which hides the older workers is not wanted.

In Norwegian: Seniorsaken (www.seniorsaken.no).

3.2. Private / commercial service enterprises

3.2.1. Vi over 60 (We over 60)

There are several providers offering services and products for seniors. One example is a weekly magazine named (in Norwegian) "Vi over 60". They offer different articles and presentations for this target group. (www.viover60.no)

3.2.2. Ressurs 50 pluss

This is an employment agency for seniors. They describe themselves as a chain between senior competence and the business field. (www.ressurs50pluss.no)

3.2.3. Internet Websites

Another group of providers develop and maintain Internet websites. Examples are:

Seniornett (www.seniornett.no) and Senior (www.senior.no).

These service enterprises offer information and help for seniors - also regarding their working life and work challenges. Due to the number of enterprises and their respective advice it is not possible to sum up their recommendations.

3.3. Research organisations

3.3.1. Norwegian Social Research (NOVA - www.nova.no)

NOVA is a research institute under the auspices of the Norwegian Ministry of Education and Research. The aim of the institute is to develop knowledge and understanding of social conditions and processes of change. It focuses on issues of life-course events, level of living conditions and aspects of life-quality as well as on programmes and services provided by the welfare system.

The institute's strategic position can be characterised as follows: "A research environment with emphasis on a broad-based social science approach combined with a life-course perspective".

3.3.2. The Work Research Institute (WRI - www.afi-wri.no)

WRI is a state-owned social science institute performing multidisciplinary, action oriented research. Its aim is to produce systematic knowledge on working life. The institute is especially concerned with forms of organisation and leadership which promote the collective ability to learn, cooperate and adapt, and thereby create a better working environment.

The institute emphasises the importance of broad, action oriented research programmes based on the needs of working life. The programmes are formed in close collaboration with Norwegian business and industry as well as with national and international research institutions. The institute also carries out shorter-term projects for organisations, companies, government agencies and other public bodies.

Most of the staff members are social scientists. The institute also benefits from the expertise provided by its graduates in engineering, law and other disciplines.

3.3.3. Fafo (www.fafo.no)

The Institute for Applied Social Science (Fafo) was founded by the Norwegian Confederation of Trade Unions in 1982. In 1993, Fafo became an independent research foundation with equity capital based on donations from the Norwegian Confederation of Trade Unions, the Norwegian Union of Municipal Employees, and several large business corporations in Norway.

The institute conducts research and studies in the fields of labour relations, welfare policy and living conditions, both nationally and internationally.

All these institutions do research in the field of elderly and older workers. The proposals of their research have been taken on board by the already mentioned organisations and have already been mentioned in this chapter.

4. Projects

4.1. Senior Revolution in the Prison Service

Oslo Prison has established a separate senior section with much success. A high degree of job satisfaction and a low absence rate are the results of this process. In addition, half the seniors want to stay on in their jobs beyond retirement age.

The senior section was established as a pilot project in 2001, and it has now become a regular feature of the prison. The youngest staff member is 48 years old.

Not only the staff and the prisoners benefit from the special section, but also the prison as a whole. The older officers possess considerable skills which no longer disappear with early retirement or long term sick leave.

Absenteeism, and especially short-term absenteeism, among the participating seniors has shown a downward trend since they were allocated their own section. For some months there has been no absence.

4.2. Better recruitment as a result of senior policy

Langerud Nursing Home is situated in Oslo. Their objective is to give the best and most comprehensive service to older people and become the best nursing home in Oslo. Three years ago a need for recruitment and reduction of costs was felt, resulting in reorganisation.

The reorganisation resulted in some new jobs for senior advisers - without a rotation system and with no overtime for elders.

Langerud strengthened their work force in two ways: by recruiting young people and at the same time keeping older and well qualified assistant nurses by offering them new and more interesting duties.

Several new arrangements were initiated. The most radical was reducing the number of nurses in the units and creating a nursing pool. Senior and well qualified assistant nurses took over their functions and were put in charge.

Another initiative in this process was the use of senior advisers. A senior adviser teaches young employees with foreign backgrounds to become care assistants. The result was that more senior assistant nurses got new job titles and new tasks.

4.3. Profitable 50-year-olds

Storebrand ASA is a Norwegian holding company with three independent business units - insurance, capital management and banking business.

Being a responsible member of society, Storebrand supports diversity and equality of status which also includes senior workers. That implies an employment policy where age has no discriminatory influence on qualifications.

Senior policy is not a matter of fashion; it is good business practice and an important issue in society. Storebrand aims to be a leading company in taking public responsibility. A definite stand on senior policy and discrimination is taken.

Some senior policy initiatives in Storebrand ASA:

- Age is of no importance, neither in recruitment nor when downsizing.
- An intranet page for presenting senior policy information.
- Personal interviews dealing with senior policy topics.
- Workers over 60 get three extra days off.
- Employees over 64 may have shorter working days than others.
- Workers past 60 get one hour physical training during the week.
- A special fund for studies has been established.

- A senior committee makes plans for altered job arrangements and retirement.
- Working from an office at home is an option.

4.4. Seniors go back to school

At *Gjøvik Trevare* (a woodworking factory) senior employees have been offered the chance to gain formal qualifications *before* the younger ones. The reason for this is that the firm places older workers on an equal footing with the younger forces and looks upon them as facilitators, role models and culture carriers.

As the seniors are the first and foremost to train the new employees it is therefore natural to give them the opportunity to obtain a craft certificate as well as their younger colleagues, according to the company's policy on seniors.

The management stresses their policy of placing seniors on an equal footing with everybody else in the firm at Gjøvik Trevare and is convinced that this will pay off.

The oldest employees pass on the firm's culture. They also have a lot of influence regarding the training activities, which is why so much attention is paid to this area. It also gives a positive signal within the company when older workers choose to spend their spare time obtaining more qualifications for their jobs.

Generally agreed are measures aimed at improving workplace environments and also address personal life-style issues. The first approach focuses on ergonomics - "setting-based actions" - while the latter focuses on personal behaviour - "behaviour-based actions". Notwithstanding this distinction these measures are strongly interconnected.

Therefore training and lectures at workplaces are given on the issue of personal life-style especially if important because of the working environment and its exposure factors. One example is particle smoke and gases from asphalt work. Smokers have a very high risk of lung disease compared to non-smokers. Therefore advice on smoke cessation is important in connection with measures to reduce exposure to hazardous substances when working.

Poland

Krzysztof Puchalski, Patrycja Wojtaszczyk

Field of promotion	Physical strain	Psyche / cognition	Mental / social competence	Professional competence
Action				
Relief of physical strain / WHP actions	Setting-based actions (ergonomics)			
Age-related working hours	Flexible retirement schemes			
Qualification				
Communication	Creating national structures for health promotion on regional and local level			
	Training of specialists for health education and promotion of training facilities			
	Development of general WHP programmes (methodology, implementation)			
	Dissemination of the national WHP concept			
	Development of supportive materials (flyers, brochures, guidebooks)			
	50+ programme (financial incentives for employers and employment offices)			
	Analysis of factors leading to unfitness to work			

* *Exercise, nutrition, consumption of alcohol and nicotine, relaxation*

Fig. 16: Summary of actions - Poland

1. Political basis

The health policy of Poland is described in two documents outlining the main objectives in the field of health. These are:

1.1. Narodowy Program Zdrowia - National Health Programme[7]

This was adopted by the government in September, 1996, and outlines the strategic goals to be realised by the Ministry of Health by 2005. The next NHP is being developed.

One of the three strategic objectives in this document is the creation of health promoting conditions for life, work and education.

This objective is to be realised mainly by reducing exposure to risk factors (part of operational goal No. 8) and reducing the number of accidents in the workplace (part of operational goal No. 10). The main outcome of this, amongst others, should be a significant drop in the number of occupational diseases (from 5 % to 50 % depending on the disease). Another important task outlined in the NHP (operational goal No. 6) is to increase the effectiveness of health education and health promotion in various settings, including workplaces, by setting up national structures on a regional and local level to give support to health promotion activities, and to develop new health education and health promotion specialists. The results are to be measured by the number of enterprises promoting health. However, the document does not specify the meaning of the term "health promoting enterprises".

The Programme shows a strong link between lifestyle, health promotion in workplaces, and a general quality of life, however, it does not cover the issue of ageing as a separate problem/challenge. The Programme is strictly a recommendation and guideline; no funds are allocated to it; its objectives are to be realised within other projects, programmes and plans.

[7] http://www.mz.gov.pl, 14.10.2004

1.2. Narodowy Plan Zdrowotny - National Health Plan[8]

The National Health Plan has been developed as a basis for the work of Ministry of Health in the field of health protection. Its creation is required under the legislation on health insurance. The plan outlines the objectives for the years 2004-2013, and was published by the Ministry on April 30, 2004. It is closely coordinated with the National Health Programme. The plan will come into force in 2005, when its objectives will be pursued. Its main objective is to reduce the number of people dying prematurely. Its goals do not include the issue of an ageing workforce as a separate field of activity. The main focuses are: cardio-vascular diseases, malignant cancer, accidents, communicable diseases, health protection for mothers and children, protracted diseases of the elderly (people over 65), mental health, rheumatism, and effectiveness of treatment. The settings approach is not included in this Plan.

2. National programmes / projects

2.1. The Ministry of Economy, Labour, Social Policy

In the years 2001-2004, a national research project concerning the professional activity of employees in the context of ageing was realised. The Ministry of Economy, Labour and Social Policy requisitioned the work performed by research institutes.

One part of it was devoted to a study of health behaviour and the development of guidelines on workplace health promotion programmes concerning ageing. The research was carried out by the Nofer Institute of Occupational Medicine. The outcomes described in PCZ 21: 21 Reports show that there are no significant differences between young and older employees as far as health awareness and health beliefs are concerned, and therefore there is no need to design separate programmes for older employees. The focus should mainly be put on developing general WHP programmes and polices that would sustain the work ability of workers during the whole of their working life and to prolong this period. Nevertheless,

[8] http://www.mz.gov.pl, 14.10.2004

methods and tools for promoting health at work have been developed since 1997 by the National Centre for Workplace Health Promotion. It is an ongoing process that includes scientific research in the field of health, health beliefs, workplace health etc. as well as the development of methodology, and the implementation of WHP programmes in particular enterprises and groups of enterprises. Additional tasks carried out are the training of specialists, the development of supportive materials and guidebooks, the dissemination of the concept and the coordination of the National Network for WHP.

In order to fight against the deficit in the state budget, a comprehensive plan has been developed by the Ministry of Economy, Labour and Social Affairs. It is a new government policy that is being introduced into Polish legislation step-by-step. A part of this plan is to enhance the work ability of older employees. But the plan also includes closely linking retirement schemes with the period of work: the longer people work, the higher the pension will be. The pension has been divided into three parts - one part is a state pension, the second an obligatory private retirement fund and the third is a voluntary private insurance.

The overall goal is to cut the amount of public money spent on early retirement benefits and pensions, and at the same time to increase the amount of money that is brought into the state budget by the taxes, premiums etc. from older employees. The solution would be to create conditions favourable for people over 45. These include more flexible retirement schemes and the "50 plus" programme (a pilot project to be introduced in 2005, aimed at the identification of labour market tools supporting the work of older employees).

This programme is in the competence of the Ministry of Economy and Labour. The pilot projects have already been accepted by the respective minister; as the call for applications for grants for this programme closed on February 14, 2005. The aim of the programme is to make it easier for people over 50 to return to work. Pilot projects include several measures: reimbursement to employers of the costs incurred by employing older workers, grants for adjusting workplaces to the needs of older workers, active training and innovative forms of work for employment offices. 20 various projects have been accepted. Each project should result in the employment of at least 50 people for six months in a non-subsidised workplace. Suggestions for effective forms of work in the future will be developed after the pilot projects have been carried out and evaluated.

2.2. The National Social Insurance Agency (ZUS)

The National Social Insurance Agency according to the respective legislation (Dziennik Ustaw 1998 No. 137, item 887) is supposed to support the prevention of occupational disability, mainly by rehabilitation and the cofinancing of research on occupational disability and accidents. They focus mostly on technical solutions in the prevention of accidents and occupational illnesses. According to the legislation concerning ZUS (Dz. U. 1998 No. 137, poz. 887, art. 66-72) this institution is entitled to conduct preventive measures concerning inability to work and rehabilitation. On the basis of that legislation they purchase medical services (mostly dental and vaccination services). Apart from that ZUS monitors and analyses the reasons for inability to work.

ZUS is also a member of the European Network of Social Insurance Institutions for Health and Work. ZUS has not yet been involved in projects concerning the ageing workforce as such; however there is an ongoing discussion about introducing instruments forcing employers to undertake more effective prevention and health promotion methods, such as social insurance premiums adjusted to the level of health risks and the number of accidents at work, related to the industry or, in the future, the enterprise.

3. Players

3.1. NGOs / interest group representatives

3.1.1. Responsible Business Forum (RBF)

The new initiative active in the field of social corporate responsibility in Poland is the Responsible Business Forum (RBF) established as an initiative of Polish businessmen, academics and NGOs. As the first of its kind in Poland, the organisation not only creates an opportunity for managers, public administration and social activists to exchange experiences, but also researches appropriate case studies in the corporate social responsibility field for enterprises acting in Poland. Responsible Business Forum is one of the first organisations in Eastern and Central Europe to promote Corporate Social Responsibility (CSR) in a comprehensive way. Since 2002, the Forum has been a national organisation partner of CSR Europe, a European network of organisations promoting Corporate Social Responsibility.[9] RBF has not yet undertaken activities concerning older employees, but it seems to be a new and potentially effective body in the field of workplace health.

3.2. Private / commercial service enterprises

Private and commercial providers of health protection and health promotion fall under no institutional monitoring concerning the content or quality of their services. Moreover there are no specific guidelines on WHP for an ageing population. The training and information on health promotion at workplaces is delivered to occupational physicians by the Institute of Occupational Medicine and also by Regional Occupational Medicine Stations (WOMP).

3.3. Research organisations

3.3.1. Nofer Institute of Occupational Medicine - The National Centre of Workplace Health Promotion

Projects on health promotion of older employees have been carried out by the Nofer Institute of Occupational Medicine - The National Centre of Workplace Health Promotion. The main focus is research.

3.3.2. Central Institute for Labour Protection - National Research Institute (CIOP - PIB)

The Central Institute for Labour Protection - National Research Institute (CIOP - PIB) conducts scientific research aimed at new technological and organisational solutions which are useful in the design of working conditions. They cooperate closely with ZUS (National Insurance Agency). Its research is oriented towards safety and ergonomics. Their guidelines are on specific factors of safety and health at work (noise, chemical substances, stress, musculo-skeletal strain etc.). The topic of ageing occurs only very rarely and no specific guidelines have been prepared yet as a result of this research.

---

[9] http://www.fob.org.pl/main/english/

4. Projects

There are no well-known examples of workplace health promotion initiatives in enterprises (apart from the research project already described) which could serve as models of good practice. However, in many WHP programmes the main focus is the prevention of illnesses that usually occur in older employees, such as breast cancer, prostate cancer, MSD etc. These are, however, general WHP programmes conducted for employees of all ages.

Romania

Theodor Haratau

<table>
<tr><th>Field of promotion</th><th>Physical strain</th><th>Psyche / cognition</th><th>Mental / social competence</th><th>Professional competence</th></tr>
<tr><td>Action</td><td></td><td></td><td></td><td></td></tr>
<tr><td>Relief of physical strain / WHP actions</td><td colspan="2">Occupational medicine examination</td><td></td><td></td></tr>
<tr><td></td><td colspan="2">Health education courses</td><td></td><td></td></tr>
<tr><td></td><td colspan="2">Counselling courses for smokers</td><td></td><td></td></tr>
<tr><td>Age-related working hours</td><td colspan="3">Accepting commuting positions (raising mobility of workforce)</td><td></td></tr>
<tr><td>Qualification</td><td colspan="4">Continuous vocational training</td></tr>
<tr><td></td><td colspan="4">Better access to highly qualified positions</td></tr>
<tr><td></td><td colspan="4">Knowledge transfer between generations</td></tr>
<tr><td>Communication</td><td colspan="4">Organisational tool to change employer's attitude towards ageing employees</td></tr>
<tr><td></td><td></td><td colspan="3">Media campaign to change general population's attitude towards ageing workforce</td></tr>
<tr><td></td><td colspan="4">Improvement of management's competences / corporate culture</td></tr>
<tr><td></td><td colspan="4">Avoidance of discriminating age-stereotypes / age-awareness culture</td></tr>
</table>

* *Exercise, nutrition, consumption of alcohol and nicotine, relaxation*

Fig. 17: Summary of actions - Romania

1. Political basis

1.1. The Ministry of Labour, Social Solidarity and Family (MMSSF)

This ministry proposes and undertakes organisational measures within the scope of statutory health and safety so as to promote Occupational Safety and Health policies. They are implemented by the ministry through its 42 Labour Inspections and their facilities. The political and financial measures of Occupational Safety and Health, proposed to promote employment policies, are implemented by the ministry through its 42 Employment Agencies within the 42 Romanian districts.

1.2. The Ministry of Health (MS)

The Ministry of Health is responsible for the elaboration and implementation of the Public Health Strategy and, as workplaces are involved, collaborates with the Ministry of Labour, Social Solidarity and Family for designing strategies and policies concerning the health of the workforce.

Through its 42 district branches, named Public Health Directorates, specific programmes in the fields of health promotion and occupational health are developed. Each District Public Health Directorate has a Health Promotion department and an Occupational Health department. Both of them deal with all the initiatives concerning workplace health promotion at district level. It has to be understood that only in the past few years have these departments started to collaborate on developing joint programmes under the topic of Workplace Health Promotion.

Both ministries, the Ministry of Labour, Social Solidarity and Family and the Ministry of Health, have jointly drafted the "Policy and strategy for Romania in the Field of Health and Safety for the Period 2004-2007".

This strategy has four main objectives, of which the third one is the following:

> "Development of activities for the prevention of work accidents and occupational diseases by forming a culture of preventing occupational risks and by an efficient combination of theoretical and practical elements."

This third objective includes other strategic objectives, specific for both of the ministries. It is of great importance to mention that among the eight objectives assigned to the Ministry of Health there is one specifically called Workplace Health Promotion which states that:

- Workplace Health Promotion activities have to be developed especially in small and medium-sized enterprises,
- these activities should aim at involving not only the employers and the employees, but the society as a whole, and
- these activities should improve general health and also consider occupational hazards.

Therefore it is worth mentioning the willingness of the Romanian stakeholders to place Workplace Health Promotion on a higher level in the political agenda and, hopefully, to assign more funds to this domain in years to follow.

1.3. The National House of Pensions and Other Social Insurance Rights (CNPAS)

It was created in 2000, and its statutes have very recently been upgraded in order to have a stronger involvement and commitment of its branches in dealing with work accidents and occupational disease insurance. A particular situation in Romania, not very often found in Europe, is that the National Fund for Accidents and Occupational Diseases (introduced by the Law 346 issued in 2002, and modified by the Government Ordinance 107/2003), has been created under the authority of this National House of Pensions. Moreover the National Institute for Medical Evaluation and Recovering of Work Capacity (introduced by the Decision of the Government No. 13 issued on January 8, 2004) has also been built under this National House of Pensions and Other Social Insurance Rights. The fact that both the Institute and the National Fund are under this Pensions House's control does not allow them to exercise autonomy in the field of promoting health and safety at work.

2. National programmes / projects

2.1. Maintaining employability for older people

The National Agency for Workforce Employment (ANOFM), a governmental agency under the Ministry of Labour, Social Solidarity and Family, launched a National Programme in 2004, with the declared scope of increasing the workforce with 189,000 persons. This national programme has eleven components, out of which two are especially targeting the ageing workforce:

- *Prolonging the active life* - offers incentives to employers hiring workers which have three years to their retirement at most. The employers receive the equivalent of the minimum wage for the industrial branch from the National Unemployment Fund for the period of employment until the retirement of the employee.
- *Diminishing long term unemployment* - a bonus-malus like initiative which is designed for those employers which hire unemployed persons over 45 years of age. The employers receive the equivalent of twelve months of minimum wage for the industrial branch from the state budget if they maintain a working contract with that person for at least two years after the first one financed by the state.

2.2 Free of charge medical assistance for elderly physicians

Starting with January 1, 2005, elderly physicians - members of the Academy for Medical Sciences, but not necessarily occupational physicians only - will receive a monthly allocation equal to the medium salary in the Romanian Economy. Medical assistance will be free of charge. The law concedes that ageing physicians can continue their work after the retirement age. By this means a limited number of physicians (hundreds) with various specialisations and a vast amount of expertise is going to remain available to the public. Those who continue to work have to be certified by the Ministry of Health and College of Physicians on an annual basis.

3. Players

3.1. NGOs / interest group representatives

3.1.1. General Assembly of the Romanian Industrialists (UGIR 1903)

The General Assembly of the Romanian Industrialists (UGIR 1903), is a confederation grouping together Associations of Employers and Professional Associations representing industry, computer technology, construction and several other economic domains, and has on its agenda the improvement of the working conditions in Romania from the employers' perspective, ageing workforce also being included.

Through several initiatives, mainly using organisational tools, this nation wide confederation is aiming to improve the employers' attitude towards the ageing workforce. In previous years, several media campaigns addressing the general population have been developed and launched with the aim of changing population's behaviour towards the older workforce. Several years ago UGIR 1903 has also organised a workshop dedicated to the ageing workforce by trying to involve several other member organisations in developing a better image of the ageing workforce by presenting various initiatives targeting this age group.

3.1.2. Bucharest Chamber of Commerce and Industry (CCIR)

The Bucharest Chamber of Commerce and Industry (CCIR), in cooperation with a German partner, initiated in 2002 a programme named "Improving Employability in Romania" which had a component concerning ageing workforce. Its aims were:

- improving the chances of ageing members of the workforce to get access to continuous training, and
- making access to skilled working positions easier for ageing members of the workforce.

The chosen method was to enhance the chances of older persons to get to better working positions by raising their professional status through training. The target has been achieved by organising training courses on topics considered to be the ones providing missing skills (project management, computer learning etc.).

3.2. Private / commercial service enterprises

3.2.1. Premier Management SRL - Modelling organisational culture

Organisational culture is one of the most decisive factors when it comes to the success of a company and, through its components, can support the process of the company's progression. Premier Management started to provide this consulting service several years ago. Its portfolio encloses companies which take into account the ageing of their entire workforce. Among the topics addressed and concerning the ageing workforce were:

- adjustments to new information technologies (i.e. vocational training),
- critical steps in accepting commuting positions (raising the mobility of the workforce), and
- coping with the "deadline style of working" (addressing the stress implied).

3.3. Research organisations

3.3.1. National Scientific Research Institute for Labour and Social Protection (INCSMPS)

The research institution with maybe the most coherent strategy towards ageing workforce is the National Scientific Research Institute for Labour and Social Protection (INCSMPS), accredited by the Ministry of Education, Research and Youth, through the Governmental Decision No. 1305 and reaccredited in 2001. Since 2000, an Excellency Centre for the labour and social protection domain has been established at the institute, according to the National Plan for Research Development and Innovation - RELANSIN Programme. The main concern of the institute is the labour and social domain. It has been targeted through research and development activities, consulting activities and scientific support activities such as research for companies/interested organisations, training, publishing a quarterly review etc.

Over the years several programmes of research have been conducted by this institute. Among the most important are:

- a study on maintaining employability for ageing workforce members,

- research on age and working capacity,
- a study on social protection for ageing workforce members, and
- a comprehensive study regarding the impact of Romania's economy, moving towards a market economy, on the ageing workforce.

3.3.2. The National Institute of Research and Development for Labour Protection (INCDPM)

The National Institute of Research and Development for Labour Protection (INCDPM) is the focal point of the Bilbao - European Agency for Safety and Health at Work and has as the main objective the development of research studies in the field of safety at work. This institute has attributions in preventing and fighting professional risks and in designing individual protection equipments. It also provides scientific background to the national institutions regulating the field of work protection and is currently developing activities of training and professional development in the field of safety at work.

3.3.3. The National Institute for Medical Evaluation and Recovery of Work Capacity

The Institute develops studies and research concerning the evaluation of working capacity and the recovery of work capacity, and therefore safety and health at work is more like an additional activity. These domains are being tackled by carrying out activities concerning the prevention of occupational diseases, health education courses, studies and research on prevention of workplace accidents, occupational orientation research and training courses, and designing programmes for disabled people.

3.3.4. The Institutes of Public Health

The Institutes of Public Health Bucharest (ISPB), Iasi, Timisoara, and Cluj, and The Centres of Public Health (Sibiu and Targu Mures) have the objective to develop research studies in the field of workplace health promotion through their Departments of Occupational Medicine and Health Promotion. It is also their task to support the Ministry of Health in elaborating strategies and policies in the domains of occupational health and safety and workplace health promotion.

3.3.5. The Institute for Research and Development in Health (INCDS)

The Institute for Research and Development in Health (INCDS) through its established National Centre for Health Promotion and Education conducts as its main task the collection and interpretation of data concerning health promotion at national level, which can contribute to the improvement of the health status of Romanian population. The National Centre for Health Promotion and Education is also responsible for the organisation of health promotion training courses for physicians and nurses.

4. Projects

4.1. Counselling courses - Selgros Romania

Selgros - a wholesaler for gastronomy and tourism - developed an extensive programme of counselling courses, tackling various topics (all health related but with emphasis on healthy working conditions), including also the ageing workforce, for which special topics have been addressed. Risk factors for older workers, healthy lifestyle - what this means for various groups and how it can be achieved -, working conditions and health, in-company medicine examinations and their importance were among the issues addressed in these courses.

Several training courses included recommendations for achieving a better health status:

- assuming an active style of life - the company supported such a lifestyle through various initiatives (supporting recurrent costs for renting sports facilities/premises, promoting transportation using bicycles, organising sport competitions etc.),
- dietary changes according to guidelines - the company produced these guidelines together with a Public Health Agency and distributed leaflets and brochures enclosing advices on how to eat in a "healthy" way,

- the company organised community based activities - increasing personal involvement in social activities (not only for the social groups at the workplace but also for the general community where the person lives), and
- "Tobacco & Health" - the company is among those trying to implement a tobacco control policy.

4.2. Tobacco and health - health education courses in Autoliv SA

In Autoliv SA - a multinational in automotive safety - the management considers smoking to be an important issue to be addressed. Accordingly, tobacco control initiatives have been developed as part of their efforts to change attitudes towards this habit. Counselling and detailed health education courses are also being developed on an ongoing basis and there is a section designed for older members of the workforce.

4.3. Expertise transfer between generations in Bere Trei Stejari SRL

The company - a brewery in Sibiu - has learned over the years that experience and expertise are gained with time and their importance in the working processes has not been receiving the proper consideration. An initiative aiming at transferring experience between generations was launched and older members of the workforce were rewarded with prizes for getting involved.

Spain

María Dolores Solé

<table>
<tr><th>Field of promotion</th><th>Physical strain</th><th>Psyche / cognition</th><th>Mental / social competence</th><th>Professional competence</th></tr>
<tr><td>Action</td><td colspan="4"></td></tr>
<tr><td>Relief of physical strain / WHP actions</td><td colspan="2">Setting-based actions</td><td></td><td></td></tr>
<tr><td></td><td colspan="2">Behaviour-based actions *</td><td></td><td></td></tr>
<tr><td></td><td colspan="2">Improvement of workplace's ergonomic design</td><td></td><td></td></tr>
<tr><td>Age-related working hours</td><td colspan="3">Part-time / flexible retirement</td><td></td></tr>
<tr><td></td><td colspan="3">Cutting daily working-hours for pre-retirees</td><td></td></tr>
<tr><td>Qualification</td><td colspan="4">Teamwork of mixed ages</td></tr>
<tr><td></td><td colspan="4">Career guidance</td></tr>
<tr><td></td><td colspan="4">Guaranteed access to continuous training / lifelong learning</td></tr>
<tr><td></td><td></td><td colspan="3">Recruitment on basis of objective criteria, i.e. avoiding age discrimination</td></tr>
<tr><td></td><td colspan="4">Adapting older workers to the changing world of work and to the requirements of new technologies</td></tr>
<tr><td>Communication</td><td colspan="4">Increasing knowledge about ergonomic problems of 50+</td></tr>
<tr><td></td><td colspan="4">Improving employability by removing barriers linked to salaries, stereotypes and continuous training</td></tr>
<tr><td></td><td colspan="4">Developing a set of quality indicators for active employment policies for a continuous control and monitoring</td></tr>
<tr><td></td><td colspan="4">Collaboration among health professionals in companies and in the national health service</td></tr>
<tr><td></td><td colspan="4">Bibliographic review on WHP measures</td></tr>
</table>

** Exercise, nutrition, consumption of alcohol and nicotine, relaxation*

Fig. 18: Summary of actions - Spain

1. Political basis

1.1. Lifelong learning

The National Foundation for Training in Employment offers financial support for vocational training. Its resources have been increased from € 763 million in 2002, to € 854 million in 2003. The percentage of workers trained who are over the age of 45 years is 18.54 %.

The recent Royal Decree 1046/2003, Order 500/2004, and the Operating Contracts Order all regulate the sub-system of continued training. Priority access to training is given to workers in SMEs (mainly less than 50 workers), women, disabled, workers over 45 years of age, and the unskilled.

1.2. Employment policies

Older people are also subject to both the National Action Plans on Employment and the National Action Plans on Social Inclusion. The Toledo Pact, signed on September 30, 2003, states the need to boost support for older workers. Limiting the use of early retirement and introducing incentives for staying on the labour market longer should serve this purpose.

A new scheme for "flexible retirement" has been set up by Law 25/2002. This new system includes:

1) Incentives for late retirement: the amount of pension is increased by 2 % for each year stayed in employment beyond the age of 65.
2) Exemptions of social security contributions for workers over 65: the present legislation on gradual and flexible retirement exempts workers aged 65 years or over from paying social security contributions if they have contributed to the system for at least 35 years.
3) Early retirement from the age of 61 years on only in exceptional cases: for people who are redundant and in real need of protection; only if they have contributed to the social security system for more than 30 years and have been unemployed for at least six months.

4) Disincentives for early retirement: reducing the pension of a worker by 6 to 8 % for each year in retirement prior to the statutory retirement age of 65.
5) Reduction in employers' social security contributions: for the age group from 60-64, companies may receive a reduction of 50 % in social security contributions for workers with seniority of at least five years. Reduction is progressively increased annually by 10 % till a complete exemption at the age of 65 is reached. Additionally, the policy to reduce social security contributions for new indefinite-term contracts for employees from the age of 45 on, initiated in 1997, is to be continued.
6) Compatibility of retirement pension (reduced accordingly) with working part-time: if the employee is between 60 and 65 years old, the company will be obliged to find a substitute by offering relief contracts to an unemployed person or a company worker with a temporary contract.
7) Redundancy for economic reasons: companies which lay off workers over the age of 55 due to economic reasons will have to pay part of these workers' social security contributions until they reach the age of 61.
8) Compatibility of unemployment benefit and salary: unemployed over 52 are entitled to receive unemployment benefit while working, with a proportional reduction in wage costs for the company recruiting them.

1.3. Social dialogue

Related to employment and equity, the process of social dialogue began in July 2004. This included the regulatory development of Organic Law 14/2003, together with support for measures promoting employment for older workers. The Organic Law 14/2003 basically governs the rights and freedoms and social integration of foreign nationals in Spain.

It includes a commitment to improving the quality of employment and promoting lifelong learning, as those active employment policies have both a qualitative and a quantitative effect. In addition, an effort will be made to integrate groups which are under-represented on the Spanish labour market at present.

Among the thirteen areas for negotiation, the ones directly related to elder workers are:

- labour market: job creation, employment stability, participation in the labour market in general and for disadvantaged groups in particular,
- knowledge-based economy: promoting lifelong learning, and ensuring occupational skills to guarantee the employability of the entire population of working age through vocational training for the unemployed, employment of social interest, career guidance, employment training, and employment for the disabled, and
- active employment policies (connected with social policies such as assistance in job-seeking, promoting employment growth, reducing unemployment) and public employment services, for example, by local development and employment specialists (PES - Public Employment Services ensuring efficacy and efficiency in questions such as information, intermediation, anticipating quantitative and qualitative employment needs, training programmes, learning and guidance, and encouraging a preventive approach), and also support for self-employment.

http://www.ilo.org/public/spanish/region/ampro/cinterfor/temas/dialogo/inf_act/dsoc_esp.pdf

1.4. Collective bargaining

An analysis of collective agreements registered during 2003, shows that 56.4 % of all salaried workers are submitted to collective agreements which include employment matters. 18 % of all these agreements (applying to 25 % of all workers) had clauses about retirement. Only a few of them include clauses for substitution contracts. Unfortunately there is no comprehensive data about health promotion for older workers.

1.5. Research funds

For the first time occupational health and safety merits a sub-programme with research funds given annually by the Ministry of Health. The aim is to promote interventions for the improvement of the quality of work. This means to improve safety and health in the workplace, create safe and healthy environments, reduce risk factors, and enhance productivity and competitiveness.

This sub-programme includes the issue "Society and Work" in which the impact of ageing is mentioned as a top priority.

As it is the first of its kind, the programme has so far only indicated the need for research on the impact of ageing on health at work, on the impact of working conditions on chronic diseases, and on rehabilitation and returning to work.

1.6. Health programmes

The strategy for public health in Spain is based on the WHO "Health for All" policy. It is the result of integrating autonomous health programmes into a unique Integrated Health Plan which gathers all the aims derived from the areas of action proposed by the WHO policy.

This plan is submitted for comments to experts and citizens. As the health programmes have to be developed each year by 17 communities of the autonomous regions the measures and interventions have to be specific and tailor-made to their present needs.

The main aims of the Plan and related activities for elder workers are currently:

Aim 5 - Ageing in good health: In 2020, people older than 65 years will have the possibility to enjoy all of their health potential and play an active social role.
Intervention: development of health policies for contributing to a sound ageing through health promotion and protection at early stages.

Aim 6 - Mental health improvement: In 2020, mental and social wellbeing will be improved and accessible and comprehensive services will be available more easily.

Intervention: work and life environment then will be designed to give people of all ages a sense of coherence, good social relationship and to empower them to be able to cope with stressful events and situations on and off the job.

Aim 13 - Health promoting arenas: In 2015, people in Spain will have more opportunities to live in a healthy social and physical environment at home, school, the workplace, and local community.

Intervention: make available mechanisms to enable people to participate in designing and improving their working and living environments, for example, in the promotion of health and wellbeing of their communities by participating in a public forum.

This general health programme is then developed by each autonomous community on the basis of practical aims and interventions.

2. National programmes / projects

2.1. National Action Plan for Employment

The following working aims have been agreed on for 2005:

- rate of employment of working people aged between 55 and 64 should rise to 41.7 %,
- increasing employment and participation in the labour market of people aged between 55 and 64, and
- measures to prolong working life - including doubling of tax credit on income for people aged 65 and beyond who decide to remain at work.

Suggestions for doing so come from the NAP itself and from social partners:

NAP:

- Promote greater adaptability of employers and employees,

- support for greater and more stable participation in the labour market,
- increase employability of every person at working age, and
- make jobs more attractive.

Government:

- Foster the modernisation of work organisation,
- invest in continuous training, R&D and ICT,
- social dialogue for analysing and revision of regulatory framework and addressing obstacles to part-time indefinite-term work,
- renew Public Employment Services and strategies: people so far receive benefits only if they take part in the employability measures proposed by the PES; in some cases, unemployment benefits may be received while an individual is also working,
- allow older people to work while receiving retirement pension,
- increase the minimum wage, and
- offer employers social security reductions in specific cases to stimulate entry and continuity in the labour market.

Unions:

- Increase employer's awareness of the problems of ageing,
- make more information available about the advantages for employers and employees about the voluntary extension of work,
- boost the programmes for age-related adaptation in SMEs; in particular the support structures for training should be organised; exchange systems between SMEs should be developed to maximise the opportunities for this age group, given the job vacancies available,
- extend continuing training of older workers, particularly in the case of the less skilled,
- establish specific programmes by the PES for older unemployed workers,
- increase labour authority vigilance in authorising redundancy plans,

- tackle age discrimination and promote the use of partial retirement measures for workers near retirement age combined with substitution contracts for young people, and
- ensure a decent minimum wage as an incentive to regular employment.

Employers:

- More extensive monitoring and evaluation by public authorities of the effect of measures taken.

2.2. Autonomous health plans (see above)

3. Players

3.1. NGOs / interest group representatives

3.1.1. Spanish Association for Standardisation and Certification (AENOR)

The Spanish Association for Standardisation and Certification (AENOR) is an independent non-profit body devoted to the development of standardisation and certification activities (S+C) in all industrial and service sectors. AENOR's aim is to contribute to the improvement of quality and competitiveness in enterprises, as well as to the protection of the environment.

At present, AENOR has about one thousand members, all of them belonging to the Spanish industrial network (natural and legal persons, public and private entities).

In its efforts to include accessibility requirements in the product and service standards addressed to the public, AENOR has approved the UNE 170006 IN report "Guidelines for standards developers to address the needs of older persons and persons with disabilities". That's why the UNE 170006 IN report was prepared in 2003, which is the Spanish translation of the CEN/CENELEC Guide 6:2002, jointly prepared by the European Committee for Standardisation CEN and the European Committee for Electrotechnical Standardisation CENELEC, which is identical to the international ISO/IEC Guide 71:2001.

3.1.2. Federació d'Associacions de Gent Gran de Catalunya (FATEC)

Catalan Federation of Old People Associations is a non profit organisation which fosters activities and actions for promoting old people and elders in society. It was created in 1982, and assembles around 500 associated members which represent 400,000 individuals. It is organised in nine territorial delegations.

FATEC has a representative member in certain bodies of Catalan Autonomous Government such as the General Committee for Social Affairs (Consell General de Serveis Socials) and the Sectorial Committee for Elderly (Consell sectorial de la Gent Gran). It's also represented at international level through FIAPA (International Federation for Elderly - see section 4.2.1.).

3.1.3. Consejo Económico y Social (CES)

The Spanish Economic and Social Council, provided for in Spain's 1978 Constitution (art. 131.2), came into being in 1991, when the law setting it up has been passed. It is a governmental advisory body that enables the economic and social partners to be involved in decisions on economic and social policy.

To be as widely accepted as possible in modern complex society, the decisions taken by the government increasingly need the participation and approval of a wide range of qualified stakeholders of social and economic interests, with the consequent benefits for governance.

The Council draws up opinions on a mandatory basis on draft bills for laws and legislative royal decrees regulating socio-economic and employment matters, and royal decrees that the government considers of particular importance in these fields. It also plays a vital role in the promotion of dialogue-leading organisations legitimately representing distinctly different interests to produce common ground and shared opinions.

Among other social topics which are directly or indirectly related to an ageing workforce, in 2000, this organisation conducted a study on the ageing workforce resulting in a set of conclusions and recommendations on retirement.

The conclusions and recommendations of the CES document occupy more than ten pages. The following are just a few of these measures:

- adapting workers to the changing world of work and to the requirements of new technologies,

- in-depth revision of current training/education proposals at all levels,
- guaranteeing the access of older workers to continuous training,
- specific and tailor-made in-house training plans,
- developing a set of quality indicators related to active employment policies for a continuous control and monitoring,
- analysing why there is only a low use of instruments related to gradual and flexible retirement and generation substitution,
- promoting good practice on redundancy plans for companies, and
- an active role for PES developing assessment and information programmes for companies, stimulating a corporate culture which allows companies to anticipate changes, and avoid drastic adaptation processes.

3.2. Private / commercial service enterprises

none

3.3. Research organisations

As the topic of ageing workforces is addressed in such various fields as sociology, technology, and innovation it is difficult to list all the research organisations dealing with the issue. And it is even more difficult to list the different projects done by them which are in some way related to ageing at work.

The web page of the collaboration among the Institute for Older Persons and Social Services (IMSERSO) and the Spanish Council for Scientific Research (CSIC) contains a who's who and a list of organisations dealing in some way with old people (and of course with ageing employees).

These websites are:
Who's who in research for elders
http://www.imsersomayores.csic.es/seniinv/index.jsp
Research Centres
http://www.imsersomayores.csic.es/seniinv/centros/index.html
Therefore two examples should be sufficient here.

3.3.1. Instituto de Biomecánica de Valencia (IBV)

IBV is a centre for R&D. Its main aim is to foster and do scientific research, technological development, technical assessment, and training in biomechanics. It was set up in 1976 by the Polytechnic University of Valencia (UPV) and the Valencia Institute of Small and Medium-Sized Enterprises IMPIVA (Institute for Valencian SMEs).

The research areas of this institute are among others: behaviour of tissues and structures of the human body; morphometry and anthropometry; evaluation of human functions and activities and industrial design, and manufacturing techniques. Some of the projects and products produced by the institute are fully applicable to old workers. Two good examples are:

- methodological procedure for designing or evaluating objects or environments for elders without disability (LONGDESIGN), and
- improvement of workplace ergonomic design for promoting healthy ageing (ERGOMAYOR).

3.3.2. National Institute for Safety and Health at Work (Instituto Nacional de Seguridad e Higiene en el Trabajo - INSHT)

The institute is, among other things, involved in the promotion and execution of activities on occupational issues. Training, information, research, study, and the dissemination of occupational risk prevention issues are its concerns. It seeks appropriate coordination and collaboration with the technical bodies involved in prevention work in each of the autonomous regions.

Related to the ageing workforce, the institute has undertaken bibliographic reviews and applied studies in companies.

At present, and as an objective for 2005, one of the groups of interest managed by INSHT - the OSH (Occupational Safety and Health) Prevention Services Network - is conducting a descriptive study on the impact of ageing among auxiliaries and nurses in some Catalan hospitals. The aim is to identify needs, collect proposals for prevention, and to promote and evaluate these measures.

4. Projects

4.1. Food and drink industry / larger company

4.1.1. HERO España

This company is a branch of Grupo HERO, a multinational in the food and drink industry sector with 730 employees and a turnover of € 182 million in 2003. From 1975, *Hero España* has adopted a strategic human resources policy aligned with a corporate culture accepted voluntarily by management and employees. It is based on the employee's personal development, team work, and the company's identification with the society where its activities take place.

The company accepts partial retirement for workers older than 60 years who want to reduce their daily work-time. This partial retirement means hiring an unemployed person to cover the remaining time and to facilitate the old worker's adaptation to and preparation for retirement.

Moreover *Hero España* has compromised on fair recruitment. Age discrimination is avoided in the areas of salaries, training, promotion, dismissal, and retirement procedures. The recruitment system is then based on objective criteria.

It also provides some social services and aid based on the social responsibility plan. For example: christmas gifts for retired workers, gifts and extra remuneration for workers with 25 or 40 years of seniority and even a journey, as well as social events for retired employees, and the like.

The positive impact of *Hero España's* human resources management together with its corporate social responsibility has been shown by the absence of labour conflicts and strikes for internal reasons over the last 25 years.

4.2. Intermediary organisations

4.2.1. Web page for elders and training course for preparing retirement

The Gent Gran website (http://www.gentgran.org/index/index8-fr.htm) is a web page in Catalan basically addressed to elders and promoted by FATEC. The web page opened on October 1, 1999, coinciding with the Day and the

International Year of the Elder. Its main aims are:

- giving access to information and resources for elders,
- opening new possibilities of participation and exchange among elders,
- showing the elder's reality and their associative reality on the web, and
- promoting access to new technologies (internet, e-mail etc.).

The Gent Gran Web page wants to be a meeting point for retirees. But it also addresses visitors who are interested in information about their own retirement or young people who look for information and services for their parents and grandparents. Among other courses (e.g. exercise for the elderly, how to get involved in the community) FATEC offers a course for citizens in transition from work to retirement. The main aim of this course is to offer information on the reorganisation of life in retirement and indicates its positive aspects. The course is structured along six main lines:

- retirement and active life,
- elders and health,
- economic aspects of retirement,
- personal development,
- interpersonal relationships, and
- active participation and social compromise.

A pedagogical kit with a textbook, two guidelines (one for individual and another for collective work) and a videotape and its guide were developed. Since 2002, they have produced more than 20 editions and trained around 500 people over 55 years.

4.2.2. ERGOMAYOR project

This project was funded by the Ministry of Labour and Social Affairs and was conducted in 2002 by IBV (see section 3.3.1.). The main objective was the improvement of working conditions for older employees.

Specific aims were to

- increase knowledge about ergonomic problems of workers older than 50 years,
- identify related factors and industrial sectors where those problems are higher,

- give recommendations on the prevention of main ergonomic problems expressed by workers, and
- establish priorities for intervention.

4.2.3. Empreses generadores de salut

Health Generating Companies (Empreses generadores de salut) is a project undertaken by the occupational health service of the Directorate General for Public Health in Valencia. This project is endorsed by the autonomous Health Ministry and is included in the health plan of this community.

The specific aims of this project are:

- providing health promotion interventions at companies,
- optimising existing WHP, and
- establishing official ways of collaboration among health professionals in companies and in the national health service.

This project is based on a comprehensive health vision: companies should participate on a voluntary basis except for mandatory interventions (level = of all proposed interventions). Participation is based on commitment and collaboration and led by health professionals.

Among the programmes included in this initiative, the following ones applied directly to old workers:

- osteoporosis,
- menopause, and
- chronic diseases.

5. Context

The coming demographic change, its economic impact on the public pension system and the number of workers needed to replace the growing number of retired workers has fostered the current reforms and interventions for old workers. It is thus a widely recognised point in Spain stressed by all stakeholders.

Nevertheless, the predictable tendency to foster the extension of the active working-life may seem contradictory in the current situation on the Spanish labour market (a high rate of inactivity and unemployment in women and lack of job security for young workers).

In order to achieve the main objective put forward for this type of measure (to reduce the burden on a social security system based on contributions) measures are also (and more frequently) stressing an improvement of the labour situation for women and young people.

General speaking, Spain has to deal with a strong demand for early retirement which began during the industrial restructuring of the 1980s, which means a continuous growth of related costs (from 4.8 % share of potential GDP in 1980 to 9.3 % in 2000, and an expected 11.1 % in 2010[10]). In the private sector the preference is still to support early retirement rather than an extension of working life. That's why strategies and policies are mainly focused on financial incentives to stay at work or retire later and to avoid an abuse of early retirement options by companies.

Current reforms as an answer to ageing in Spain mainly involve

- new systems for access to retirement called "flexible retirement". This reform has taken place at social partner level and is based upon personal decision to retire. The aim is to facilitate a progressive transition from work to retirement instead of a sharp interruption.
- Measures to foster the demand for older workers (e.g. reducing or waiving social security contributions).
- Incentives to remain at work (disincentives for leaving work).
- Improving employability of older workers by removing barriers linked to salaries, stereotypes and continuous training (quantity and quality).

[10] Herbertsson, T.T; Orszag, J.M. The early retirement burden: Assessing the costs of the continued prevalence of early retirement in the OECD countries. IZA DP 816 Bonn (2003)

Sweden

Bo Hagström, Ewa Menckel

<table>
<tr><th>Field of promotion</th><th>Physical strain</th><th>Psyche / cognition</th><th>Mental / social competence</th><th>Professional competence</th></tr>
<tr><td>Action</td><td colspan="4"></td></tr>
<tr><td>Relief of physical strain / WHP actions</td><td colspan="4">Job task exchange</td></tr>
<tr><td></td><td colspan="2">Behaviour-based actions *</td><td></td><td></td></tr>
<tr><td></td><td colspan="3">"Plus All" - physical activities during paid working hours (e.g. nursing staff)</td><td></td></tr>
<tr><td></td><td colspan="3">Effective management systems</td><td></td></tr>
<tr><td></td><td colspan="3">Good working environment</td><td></td></tr>
<tr><td></td><td colspan="4">Setting up special departments for senior workforce</td></tr>
<tr><td></td><td colspan="3">Accepting help from other workers with difficult work task (e.g. lifting heavy weights)</td><td></td></tr>
<tr><td></td><td colspan="3">Reducing working hours in favour of other occupational tasks (e.g. teachers)</td><td></td></tr>
<tr><td>Age-related working hours</td><td colspan="2">Flexible working hours for ageing workforce</td><td></td><td></td></tr>
<tr><td></td><td colspan="3">Reducing working hours at advanced age</td><td></td></tr>
<tr><td>Qualification</td><td colspan="4">"Activity Guarantee" - continued vocational training</td></tr>
<tr><td></td><td colspan="4">"Knowledge Lift" - adult education</td></tr>
<tr><td></td><td colspan="4">"Knowledge Diffusion" - aka mentorship</td></tr>
<tr><td></td><td colspan="4">Installing "Resource Units" - staff pool to handle short-time absence (e.g. hospitals)</td></tr>
<tr><td></td><td colspan="4">Lifelong learning opportunities</td></tr>
<tr><td></td><td colspan="4">Personal "Educational Savings Accounts" - a government competence bonus</td></tr>
</table>

Field of promotion	Physical strain	Psyche / cognition	Mental / social competence	Professional competence
Communication	Abolishing prejudices towards ageing workforce			
	Good leadership			
	Career counselling			

** Exercise, nutrition, consumption of alcohol and nicotine, relaxation*

Fig. 19: Summary of actions - Sweden

1. Political basis

1.1. Swedish Work Environment Authority (Arbetsmiljöverket, AV)

The paramount objective of AV is to reduce the risks of ill-health and accidents at the workplace and to improve overall working environments in a holistic perspective, i.e. from a physical, mental, social, and organisational point of view.

1.2. Swedish National Labour Market Administration (Arbetsmarknadsverket, AMV)

The Swedish Labour Market Administration is responsible for translating Swedish labour market policy into practice. The central authority of the Swedish Labour Market Administration is the National Labour Market Board. In each of Sweden's 21 counties there is a County Labour Board, to which the Public Employment Services are responsible.

1.3. Insurance Office (Försäkringskassan)

The role of the Insurance Office is to administer social insurance and to ensure that people obtain the benefits and allowances which they are entitled to. To be covered by or to be eligible for such benefits, one must, as a rule, either be resident in Sweden or be working here. Examples of residence-based benefits are child allowance, housing allowance and allowance for medical expenses. There is a regional office in every Swedish county with totally 240 local offices. The total workforce consists of 16,000 people. The head office is located in Stockholm.

1.4. The National Board of Health and Welfare (Socialstyrelsen, SoS)

SoS is a national expert and supervision authority concerning social work (child-care, care of elderly, and care of individuals and families as well as addicts), health and safety, contagious diseases, and health and medical care. SoS works to ensure that measures in these fields are of high quality and distributed according to requirements. SoS can be seen as a supervisory and advisory governmental authority of the Swedish welfare system.

1.5. The National Institute of Public Health (Folkhälsoinstitutet, FHI)

FHI in Sweden is a national centre of excellence for the development and dissemination of methods and strategies in the field of public health. It is responsible for the comprehensive cross-sectoral follow-up and evaluation of national public health policy and exercises supervision in the areas of alcohol, drugs and tobacco abuse. Activities are conducted on the basis of scientific evidence.

1.6. The Development Council for the Government Sector (Utvecklingsrådet för den statliga sektorn)

The purpose of the Council is to facilitate local development measures in the form of financial support, to arrange working networks between government institutions, provide guidelines and books, arrange seminars and conferences etc. All the activities are based on the cooperation between the social partners, at local and at national level. Representatives of employers' and employees' organisations form steering committees and work together in national and local projects. The Council provides funds for project management, documentation and evaluation; the local institutions usually provide resources of their own to participate in the development projects.

1.7. Occupational Health and Safety, OHS (Företagshälsovården, FHV)

The employer should guarantee the existence of an available OHS according to working conditions (SFS 1977:1160 § 2 b). OHS in the Swedish context means an independent expert resource in the field of working environment and rehabilitation. In particular, the OHS is supposed to prevent and remove health hazards at the workplace, and to identify and describe the connections between work environment, organisation, productivity and health (SFS 1999:841).

2. National programmes / projects

2.1. Aktivitetsgarantin (the "Activity Guarantee")

As part of the Swedish active labour market policy a so called activity guarantee (aktivitetsgaranti) has been introduced for people who are or run the risk of being long-term unemployed - among them a substantial number of elderly people. The aim of this guarantee is to offer unemployed persons new opportunities to enter the labour market, to prevent their elimination, and thereby increase the supply of labour.

The activity guarantee means either full-time activities up to employment on the open labour market or training in the ordinary education system. This way of working provides the opportunity to support the applicant's endeavours to get a job in a more concentrated way through organised job-finding activities or by offering vocational training courses, practical experience or different forms of employment support. Because of how it is constructed the activity guarantee prevents the improper use of unemployment insurance as a financial supplement while waiting for retirement.

2.2. Kunskapslyftet (the "Knowledge Lift")

In recent years Sweden carried out a great venture in adult education to raise the level of knowledge. Within the scope of this so called Kunskapslyftet, between 1997-2002, roughly 800,000 people were given access to such an education. In this way, life-long learning has been widespread - especially among elderly persons.

2.3. Näringsdepartementets seniorgrupp

In 2001, the Ministry of Industry, Employment and Communication appointed a group, "The Senior Group" (Näringsdepartementets seniorgrupp), with the purpose of identifying existing obstacles in agreements and legislation concerning the possibility for elderly people to remain on the labour market. If necessary, the group was expected to suggest changes in the present status. The group delivered its final report in 2002 (Riv hindren för äldre i arbetslivet, Ds. 2002:10) with a number of suggestions to make it easier for elderly people to remain an active part of working life. Some of these proposals were:

- A more generous attitude towards a longer absence for trying another job might be an alternative, in order to increase personal job-mobility.
- The Swedish payroll tax for employees older than 65 should decrease further.
- Education and competence development should be assisted. Vocational training courses need to be adjusted to the needs of elders: special pedagogical methods need to be developed and enterprises ought to develop and systematise their internal training especially for elders and/or employees with a low level of education.
- The government ought to participate in improving adult pedagogy and also create a form of study finance which functions well and so facilitates job change for adults.
- Personal "educational savings accounts" ought to be introduced which all individuals can use. When somebody withdraws a specific amount from this account to finance the development of their skills and competence, a government competence bonus should be granted related to the extent of the competence development.
- Switch-over positions from manager/director to administrator/civil servant need to be played down. Some top positions ought to have a time-limit in order to stimulate turnover at the top level.

2.4. "Age and Working Life"

In autumn 2001, the Development Council for the Government Sector started the project "Age and Working Life". Demographic development suggests there may be a manpower shortage in future - especially among well-trained workers. The problem is reinforced by the fact that older members of the workforce have a tendency to leave working life many years before statutory retirement age.

The long-term aims of the project "Age and Working Life" was to contribute to solving the government's problem of maintaining competence, partly because elderly employees both want to and are able to work longer, partly by attracting younger employees. This can be done by creating an attractive working life with a good working environment, stimulating work, flexible working hours, good leadership, effective management systems and other appropriate methods, models and tools. In dialogue with a great number of authorities the project has analysed the need for action through, for example, dialogue seminars at different places in Sweden. The seminars have been documented in order to disseminate ideas and to serve as sources of inspiration for the authorities in their work.

3. Players

3.1. NGOs / interest group representatives

3.1.1. National social partners

Swedish Agency for Government Employers (SAV), The Swedish Association of Local Authorities and Regions (SALAR), Federation of Swedish Enterprises (SN), Federation of Private Enterprises, Swedish Trade Union Federation (LO), Swedish White Collar Trade Union Confederation (TCO), Swedish Confederation of Professional Associations (SACO).

3.1.2. Swedish Occupational Health and Safety Association (Föreningen Svensk Företagshälsovård, FSF)

FSF, as a member organisation for the Swedish Occupational Health and Safety organisations, aims at working for development in the areas of work environment and work-related rehabilitation. The bottom line is also to represent the branch by pointing out the advantages of the OHS to the parliament and the government, authorities, social partners and enterprises. Today OHS is established all over Sweden and consists of approximately 750 units. OHS acts as a resource on work environment issues for enterprises, organisations and the public sector. OHS employs approximately 7,000 staff, mainly with medical, technical and psychological competence.

3.2. Private / commercial service enterprises

3.2.1. AFA Insurance

AFA is the umbrella organisation for life insurance, group health insurance and no-fault liability insurance. Its main objective is to administer insurances which are stipulated in collective agreements or other agreements between social partners. The insurances are valid for shortage of work, illness, parental leave, occupational injury and death. Approximately 3 million people are served by at least one of these insurances. That makes each company within AFA the biggest insurance company in this area. AFA also arranges and carries out education about insurances.

3.3. Research organisations

3.3.1. The National Institute for Working Life (NIWL)

The National Institute for Working Life (NIWL) is Sweden's national centre of knowledge for all issues concerning working life and conducts its research and development activities on commission of the Ministry of Industry, Employment and Communications. The Institute is residing in different regions of Sweden, the head office being in Stockholm.

There are eight main areas of research and development:

- health and ill-health in working life,
- the labour market and employment,
- work organisation,
- ergonomics and work load,
- labour legislation in transformation,
- integration and diversification,
- physical and chemical health hazards, and
- development processes in working life.

Research is multidisciplinary and arises from problems and trends in working life; communication and information being an important aspect of the work. The programmes or projects have been conducted either in cooperation with other institutes and universities or through collaboration between researchers inside the Institute itself.

Of particular relevance are topics such as ageing and the ageing workforce. Five examples are given in section 4. (www.niwl.se)

3.3.2. The National Institute of Public Health (Folkhälsoinstitutet, FHI)

FHI is a national centre of excellence in Sweden for the development and dissemination of methods and strategies in the field of public health, and is responsible for comprehensive cross-sectoral follow-ups and evaluation of national public health policies. It exercises supervision in the areas of alcohol, drugs and tobacco. The activities are conducted on the basis of scientific evidence. FHI normally works at national level with information, conferences, seminars, good practice dissemination etc.

3.3.3. Swedish Council for Working Life and Social Research, (FAS)

The Council's main support for research is giving grants for projects. To stimulate research within specific areas the Council may award longer-term grants to research programmes at academic departments of excellence. The council also institutes research positions at Swedish universities and provides grants for visiting researchers as well as scholarships for post-doc studies abroad.

The research which is funded by the Council covers, for example, chemical and physical hazards at work, including electromagnetic fields, stress, work and health, work organisation, labour market issues, public health and health services, elders and disability. Of particular interest is multidisciplinary research and research that addresses topics relating to equality between the sexes.

As it is an important national governmental council, occupied with the research funding of Working Life research and Social research, FAS is very important for the WHP work in Sweden; however, making explicit suggestions on WHP measures does not lie within its portfolio.

3.3.4. Swedish Institute for Social Research (Institutet för social forskning, SOFI, Stockholm University)

SOFI was established 1972 as part of Stockholm university. SOFI does research concerning social labour market issues. At SOFI there are professorships in the following: labour market policy, economics with a special focus on evaluating labour market research, sociology focusing on social politics, sociology especially focusing on unemployment and marginalisation and two professorships in sociology with a special focus on levels of living standards. SOFI has a staff of about 60 employees.

3.3.5. Statistics Sweden (Statistiska Centralbyrån, SCB)

Statistics Sweden is a central government authority for official statistics and other government statistics, and in this capacity also has the responsibility for coordinating and supporting the Swedish system for official statistics. Being the main source of national statistical data it hence also becomes the main source for Swedish working life researchers.

3.3.6. All Swedish universities and university colleges

All Swedish universities and university colleges have faculties - or at least studies - concerning working life.

4. Projects

4.1. Research programme - "Work after 45"

The title of the programme was "Work after 45 - A National Programme about the Ageing of the Workforce in Sweden". This multidisciplinary programme was implemented at the National Institute for Working Life (NIWL - see 3.3.1.) from 1990 to 1996, and ended with both the international scientific conference "WORK AFTER 45?" and the publication of a textbook (in Swedish) "Arbete efter 45" (Work after 45 - historical, psychological and physiological perspectives on ageing in work-life). The overall aim of the programme was to develop knowledge benefiting health, commitment to work, productivity and personal development of 45+ age groups.

The larger studies focused on:

- Musculoskeletal functions and disorders: the results suggest implications for career counselling and show the importance of continuous competence development that enables elderly workers to change to physically less demanding jobs.
- Early retirement: the study shows that risk factors up to eight years before exit were:
    - social: unemployment, divorce, immigrant status;

    - work-related: repetitive and monotonous work, heavy manual handling. No obvious gender differences in risk factor patterns were identified, however, high age (above 60) was a strong risk factor.
- Middle-aged and elderly employees' ability to cope with downsizing: ill health resulting from coping with downsizing was predominantly caused by previous existing health problems, but can also be exacerbated by threatening life situations.
- A conclusion from the study on middle-aged and elderly home carers' capacity to combine mental and physical demands in their work is that the demands should be decreased. They should also been given support because many of them experience feelings of insufficiency and insoluble conflicting demands.

The influence of various kinds of reorganisation on young and older employees was also investigated.

4.2. Research programme - "Ageing and Occupational Accidents"

The programme had the overall title "Ageing and Occupational Accidents - a longitudinal analysis of age-related risk patterns as a basis for targeted occupational-accident prevention and a general methodology for utilising data registers in injury prevention". The programme was implemented in collaboration of Karolinska Institutet and the NIWL (see 3.3.1.). It investigated age-related processes by studying accident hazards in four targeted occupations (miners, assemblers, nurses, and hospital auxiliaries). On the basis of national accident registers, the occupations were studied one at a time, separately for men and women. Accident risks (encompassing frequency, severity and characteristics of injuries) were investigated longitudinally: by age category, across age categories, and by cohort.

The review of the literature of the last three decades does suggest that workers of different ages are susceptible to different kinds of injuries.

In general, it seems that older workers have lower accident ratios but one of the explanations could be lower risk exposure. For safety reasons and prevention there is a need to pay greater attention to the accident risk distribution across age categories - better surveys of accidents together with expert groups could be a suggestion.

The workers themselves could increase their physical ability and accept help more often from other workers to deal with a work task. The manager could give the workers better ways to reduce lifting and "hard" work tasks, and give opportunities for changing or reducing work tasks or work hours. The personnel at the occupational health services could give advice and information.

4.3. Work after 45 - conclusions from a research programme

The National Institute for Working Life (NIWL) summarised knowledge and experiences of ageing and an ageing workforce in a popular scientific publication in 2003 (in Swedish). The publication was based on interviews with some of the researchers who contributed to the textbook mentioned above, namely "Work after 45". The interviews show that the questions posed in 1990 were still relevant, but that new knowledge and perspectives have been developed since then. The publication covers areas such as the elderly at work in a historical perspective, attitudes towards the elderly, the demands for adaptation imposed by a longer working life, preventive interventions as the best remedy, ageing and memory, facts and prejudices about the elderly, age and job performance, lifelong learning opportunities, the need for capacity to meet demands and risks in an ever tougher work climate, and the voice of free will as the most important factor.

4.4. Intervention programme for older school teachers

In Malmö Municipality, the third largest municipality in Sweden, an intervention programme for older teachers was initiated in 1998. The background to this was the fact that the municipality had problems in recruiting new teachers and in retaining the services of older teachers, especially at compulsory-school level.

Three projects were initiated. It was the third, however, called "Action for the enabling of older teachers" that was most appreciated and received the most attention. So far, it has encompassed around 100 teachers. They have obtained reduced teaching time in exchange for other tasks, such as library duties, IT, working on the curriculum, dealing with cultural issues, and being involved in matters of mentorship and school development.

The programme has had a positive impact on personnel policy in Malmö City. The "Action for the enabling of older teachers" project continues, whereas the other two have been discontinued. Up to and including 2005, a total of SEK 100.5 million has been allocated to the programme, which is regarded as money well employed. Currently, there is no shortage of teachers in Malmö City, and older teachers are secure in the knowledge that opportunities for both support and other work tasks are available.

4.5. Good practices for promoting continuous working life for elderly

This project, which is based on a self-reporting survey of 3,000 health care personnel in Region Skane in southern Sweden, embraces a mapping of "Good Examples" that promote a continuous working life among elderly workers. The highlighted examples in this study are *"resource units"*, *"knowledge diffusion"*, *"job task exchange"* and *"health promotion"*.

"Resource units" are an alternative for those people with good self-confidence and competence to have the courage to go on working and try something new. The resource units are a kind of staff pool to handle short-time absences at the hospital, which need experienced personnel. They report that in this way working at the resource units prolongs their working life.

"Knowledge diffusion" gives the older employees more acknowledgement and significance. It makes working life more interesting and for this reason can extend working life.

"Job task exchange" helps the elderly worker to deal with their job in a better way, either in order to prevent monotony or to facilitate work. A job task exchange can also reduce the risk of "being locked up". This means that less anxiety evolves among employees, as reorganising work can exert a positive effect and is an appeal to continue working.

"Health promotion" is a way to help elderly workers to attain better health - another way to extend working life.

"Plus All" is a health promotion project that could serve as an example: within the home help service, nursing staff are offered 3 and 2 hours/week of

so-called "quality time" during paid working hours. 78 % of the personnel say that their desire to remain working in the home help service has increased. The physical activities chosen are fitness training, jogging, and massage.

The conclusion seems to be that all the practices mentioned can give positive support for an extended working life. But there is no scheme that would suit everyone; the solutions have to be tailor-made.

4.6. Senior department at the prison in Gothenburg

The aim is to set up a special department for elderly personnel where work is adjusted to allow them to remain at work until statutory retirement age, with good health, lower absence due to illness and good work satisfaction. Furthermore, the department will make use of the solid professional experience of the elderly. As mentors they will transfer knowledge to the younger colleagues, who work at the department as "disciples". The target group for getting work at the senior department are employees at the KVS (Kriminalvårdsstyrelsen, The Prison and Probation Administration) who are older than 50. The target group for the mentor activities are those who have been employed relatively recently and who need to be strengthened in their professional role.

Switzerland

Joseph Weiss

<table>
<tr><th>Field of promotion</th><th>Physical strain</th><th>Psyche / cognition</th><th>Mental / social competence</th><th>Professional competence</th></tr>
<tr><td>Action</td><td></td><td></td><td></td><td></td></tr>
<tr><td>Relief of physical strain / WHP actions</td><td colspan="2">Workplace health promotion measures *</td><td></td><td></td></tr>
<tr><td></td><td colspan="4">New forms of task for ageing workers (coaching, consulting etc.)</td></tr>
<tr><td></td><td colspan="3">Use of work ability index</td><td></td></tr>
<tr><td>Age-related working hours</td><td colspan="2">Flexible working hours linked to age</td><td></td><td></td></tr>
<tr><td></td><td colspan="2">Individual organisation of working hours</td><td></td><td></td></tr>
<tr><td></td><td colspan="2">Age-related part time work</td><td></td><td></td></tr>
<tr><td></td><td colspan="2">Flexible pension / retirement entry model</td><td></td><td></td></tr>
<tr><td></td><td colspan="3">Reduction of working hours instead of dismissals when downsizing</td><td></td></tr>
<tr><td>Qualification</td><td></td><td colspan="3">Continuous further training</td></tr>
<tr><td></td><td></td><td colspan="3">Age-friendly learning</td></tr>
<tr><td></td><td colspan="4">Agreement on goals</td></tr>
<tr><td></td><td colspan="4">Career planning</td></tr>
<tr><td></td><td colspan="4">Flexibility on the labour market (job rotation etc.)</td></tr>
<tr><td></td><td colspan="3">Personal flexibility of the worker (type of job, place of work)</td><td></td></tr>
<tr><td>Communication</td><td colspan="3">Basic course on health and work ability</td><td></td></tr>
<tr><td></td><td colspan="4">Adequate age diversity / generation mix</td></tr>
</table>

Field of promotion	Physical strain	Psyche / cognition	Mental / social competence	Professional competence
	Improved social competence of managers towards older workers			
	Employer contributes to content and financing of further training programme			
	Further training can be consumed during working hours			

** Exercise, nutrition, consumption of alcohol and nicotine, relaxation*

Fig. 20: Summary of actions - Switzerland

1. Political basis

Federal council report on legislative planning for 2003-2007

The Swiss Federal Council wants older workers to be integrated in the work process both better and longer than is the case today. A suitable policy has to be developed, which will be supported and carried out at every level of the state and by the social partners. On the basis of a study, the Federal Council will decide whether legislation is needed to eliminate the discrimination of older workers on the labour market and to promote and encourage their employment.

A wide range of measures are to be tested:

- health protection at the workplace,
- ergonomic and organisational adaptations at the workplace for older workers,
- greater choice of working hours and age-related part-time work, and
- more focus on further training.

Results will show which measures will have to be taken by companies and which measures should be allocated to the social partners, and also what labour regulations or other state measures are necessary. At the end of the year, the Federal Council will receive a report giving recommendations for measures concerning social insurance, employability on the labour market, and health and work.

1.1. State Secretariat for Economic Affairs (seco)

Seco is the centre of competence of the federal government for all central questions of economic policy. Seco's aim is to create a framework of order and economic policy so that the economy can develop for the benefit of all. In domestic affairs, seco is the interface between business, the social partners and politics. It also monitors health and safety at workplace at federal level.

1.1.1. Economic growth report

In seco's economic growth report, one of the aims it sets is the maintenance of a high volume of work and the increase of productivity. To maintain a high degree of participation on the labour market, labour market flexibility (good health, polyvalent training and experience, flexibility regarding place of work etc.) should be ensured and incentives should be created to encourage older workers to be more mobile.

1.2. Federal Office of Public Health (BAG)

BAG makes an essential contribution towards keeping the population in good health. It measures its success by the effect on public health.

1.3. Federal Social Insurance Office (BSV)

The BSV is the federal competence centre for issues concerning old age, invalidity and the family. It plans, guides and monitors the respective social insurance systems to ensure they function correctly. Additionally, it coordinates reciprocal social insurance agreements with other countries.

In 2003, the BSV published a report "Workplace policy in practice in the nineties and perspectives" in which areas for the employment of older workers were identified and various measures for their promotion were suggested. These recommendations to the older members of the workforce and their employers apply to the periodic talks on qualifications and goals. An assessment of personal ability should be the basis for a medium-term career plan and a short-term agreement of goals (generally for one year). The career plan should include the development of the worker (work portfolio, position in the hierarchy, working hours, further training, and the date and form of retirement, if this is intended in the next 3-5 years).

1.4. Federal Statistical Office (BFS)

This is the federal centre of competence for official statistics in Switzerland. It steers and co-ordinates the statistics at all levels - federal, canton and municipality - and is the centre which monitors the condition and development of the population, the economy, society, land and environment in Switzerland.

1.4.1. Swiss Labour Force Survey (SAKE)

Each year a survey is carried out by order of the Federal Council to collect data on the labour market and working life in general, as well as on special groups - including older persons. In 2002, the results showed that every second person retired before reaching retirement age, and that 40 % of these retirements were for health reasons or because of company reorganisation.

1.4.2. Swiss Health Survey

At regular intervals, a survey is carried out which gives a reliable picture of the general health of all age groups in the population. It is based on the personal assessment of individual health.

1.4.3. Swiss Health Observatory (OBSAN)

OBSAN is a federal and cantonal institution which processes and analyses available health data in Switzerland. It provides support for the federal government, the cantons and other health service institutions in their planning, decision-making and actions. Through its analyses and reports, OBSAN plays a part in providing a knowledge-based health service in Switzerland.

1.5. State Secretariat for Education and Research (BBW)

The BBW is the federal authority for national and international issues concerning general and university education and research. It prepares and implements the federal policy on science, research, universities and education.

1.6. Federal Office for Professional Education and Technology (BBT)

BBT is the federal centre of competence for issues concerning vocational training, including the health service, universities of applied science and innovation policy.

2. National programmes / projects

2.1. State Secretariat for Economic Affairs (seco)

Project "Participation of older workers on the labour market"

The steering group responsible for implementing the goals of the Federal Council for 2005 in "Report on measures promoting the labour market participation of older workers" set up three working groups. There will be a report on this issue from each of three different perspectives: social insurance, employability, and health and working conditions.

The report on "Health and Working Conditions" should contain a catalogue of proposals for measures describing how to enable workers to take an active role in working life. Another aspect of working conditions and health protection being studied is how to eliminate incentives which encourage workers to take early retirement.

The measures themselves should help older workers to stay at work and promote their ability to work. The results of the measures will affect companies and the social partners, will cause changes in laws, or will be realised at Federal Council or administrative level. Information on the measures developed can only be given when the report has been presented to the Federal Council.

2.2. Federal Office for Social Security (BSV)

The continuous revision of the invalidity insurance law envisions an innovation in the form of systematic early diagnosis, for the time being within the scope of a project. The monitoring and integration of all persons who are unable to work because of illness will be carried out.

2.3. State Secretariat for Economic Affairs (seco) and Health Promotion Switzerland (foundation)

The National Conference for Workplace Health Promotion 2005, entitled "40plus - Health and experience as company potential" took place on March 16, 2005, in the University of Bern. The issue was the ageing of our society and its effects on working life. By seeing examples of good practice, enterprises should be motivated to take early steps to retain the work ability, motivation and health of their employees. The target participants are personnel experts and health representatives in companies. Over 420 people attended the conference, which was a complete success according to the feedback. All the contributions are available at www.bgf-tagung.ch.

3. Players

3.1. NGOs / interest group representatives

3.1.1. Health Promotion Switzerland (foundation)

The aims of Health Promotion Switzerland are to ensure that:

- health promotion has an obvious place on the agenda of Swiss policy and also that it is well accepted by the general public, and
- health promotion is at a very high professional standard when compared internationally, and that good ideas are implemented efficiently in effective projects.

Information is available at www.gesundheitsfoerderung.ch

3.1.2. Swiss Association for Workplace Health Promotion

The Swiss Association for Workplace Health Promotion was founded in 2003 under the patronage of the State Secretariat for Economic Affairs (seco). Private enterprises founded it as an association. Its purpose is to provide the opportunity for the exchange of experience and knowledge between its members and the development of mutual activities for workplace health promotion (WHP) as a corporate policy and part of the corporate culture. At present, the association holds a so-called ERFA-day (exchange of experience = ERFahrungsAustausch). Experts are invited to provide contributions on special topics, and models of good practice in companies are presented and discussed. Information is available at www.svbgf.ch and in its member section are tools for age management in the enterprises.

3.1.3. Pro Senectute

Pro Senectute gives advice to older people and their relatives. In politics, it campaigns for good solutions which favour elders. A course informs about all the important aspects concerning imminent retirement, such as health and vitality, financial and personal security, changes in everyday life, changes in the network of relationships, ideas for new activities, a glimpse of the manifold opportunities in sports, education and entertainment.

3.1.4. Network for Socially Responsible Business (NSW-RSE)

NSW-RSE is an association consisting of citizens, enterprises and non-profit organisations. Their aim is to influence the development of business in the age of globalisation for the benefit of everyone concerned. A project realised with the aid of the Zurich Society for Human Resource Management, "The employment of ageing staff members: problems and solutions" ended with the publication of the book "Older people at work" (Ältere Menschen im Unternehmen) in 2004. On the last page of the book there are twelve recommendations to companies and politicians:

1) Age is not a good selection criterion.
2) Learning must be suited to age.
3) The person is important, not the age.
4) Don't rely on tests which have little significance.
5) Ensure a good diversity of ages.
6) Good training and good health are essential requirements.
7) Don't forget that knowledge is stored in human heads.
8) Retain work ability and employability.
9) Remember that the employment contract also has a psychological factor.
10) Be careful with specialisation.
11) Suitable payment and personnel policy.
12) Attitude is decisive.

3.2. Private / commercial service enterprises

3.2.1. Private and semi-private advisory services

3.2.1.1. AEH Zentrum GmbH

When designing workplaces, AEH takes the physical requirements of older people into consideration, particularly regarding visual tasks and motoric activities. The work ability index is used for occupational medical examinations and for assessments in company case management. Two courses are being developed, one for persons directly affected and one for human resource personnel.

3.2.1.2. Institut Universitaire Romand de Santé au Travail (IST - foundation)

This research institute also offers services in the field of occupational medicine, hygiene, psychology and ergonomics. Its planned project "Health and work at the age of 50 and more: favourable work environment to physical and mental health" will contain a study on the international literature and several seminars for stakeholders at cantonal level. The enterprises concerned should try to keep their workers healthy by using setting-oriented measures so that they are able to work longer. The "Work Ability Index" is used in this project.

3.2.1.3. Movis AG

Workplace social consultancy is the core business of Movis, and health is an important issue.

The seminars they offer under the titles "Perspectives 45+" and "45+ - A management task" provide support for successful in-house policy on ageing. Management and staff learn the basics on well-being and work ability, the phase of life starting at 45, and work-life balance.

They can deal with the coming phase in their life and job and develop realistic perspectives for their career and the retention of their ability to work.

3.2.1.4. Hochschule für Sozialarbeit (HSA) Bern

In the post graduate course "Ageing - life design 50+" the students gain qualifications which enable them to take on challenging tasks in planning, project leadership, policy development, setting up services and infrastructure, training, advising and marketing for people of middle age and above.

3.3. Research organisations

3.3.1. Zürcher Hochschule Winterthur ZHW - Results of research on workplace ageing policies

A study is being carried out to find out what strategies Swiss companies used in the nineties and what conditions influenced early retirement. The study should lead to a typology of the enterprises according to how they deal with persons approaching retirement. 120 enterprises and 170 employees were studied. The following results and recommendations can be found in the report "Workplace policy in practice in the nineties and perspectives - research report No. 4/03" (http://www.bsv.admin.ch/aktuell/presse/petersinsel/d/4_03_eBericht.pdf):

- Individual organisation of working hours
- Age-linked working hours
- New kinds of employment for older workers (coaching, consulting etc.)
- Reduction of working hours instead of dismissals when downsizing
- Continuing general further training
- Flexible retirement entry
- Increased personal flexibility for the employee (job, place of work, working hours, job rotation)
- Employer contributes to the content and financing of further training programmes
- Time off to attend further training programmes
- Improved social competence for management when dealing with older workers
- Age diversity

Additionally, as a result two basic proposals for ageing-friendly employment were formulated (Report p. 107 ff.):

"(7) The employability of members of the workforce from between 45 to 50 can primarily be retained by promoting the qualification, motivation, personal initiative and mobility of the older workers and by offering and using flexible models of working and new working conditions (content, function, role).

(8) A central requirement in the transition period for older workers of 60 and above is a flexible model of retirement and new forms of employment (work content, functions, roles) which enable a smooth exit from working life."

4. Projects

4.1. Industry

4.1.1. ABB Switzerland

The company deals with the issue of older workers through the implementation of their strategy and various offers. At present, the personnel management is working on a new sustainable policy "Older Workers at ABB Switzerland".

Currently, ABB is especially promoting the chance to take flexible retirement and workers frequently take advantage of this. Moreover, at the age of 60, all the members of higher management transfer to ABB Consulting, which is run as an independent company and offers internal and external consultancy services. The aim is to enable knowledge to be passed on from the older employees to the younger ones, and to offer the younger ones the opportunity of promotion.

4.2. Retail

4.2.1. Migros Genossenschafts-Bund

The project "Midlife Power Programme (MPP)" especially concerns the age group of the 40-50-year-olds in the company who want have at least another 15 years of working life full of energy, as well as the parts of the company which have recognised this potential and would like to use it.

In November 2001, a training module was introduced in order to motivate and encourage the 45-50-year old employees. The aim of the programme was to utilise the potential of this age group, increase their employability, and bind the long-serving employees to the company. This increases competitive advantage.

A particular goal of the programme is to create a new awareness of the qualities of this age group and to reduce any possible feeling of resignation. The programme includes a personal assessment, workshops on special issues, and innovation circles. It is highly valued by the participants and has already had results (e.g. increased self-confidence, reduction of working hours, participation in new training courses). As an effect of the positive results, Migros intends to offer the programme again and to make it more widely available.

4.2.2. Genossenschaft Migros Zurich

Lighter work with easier conditions was created for older, less able workers within the scope of a short-term project. The measures were evaluated regarding their cost effectiveness. Ergonomic factors in workplace design were especially considered and technical aids to relieve physical strain were provided.

4.3. Social Services

4.3.1. Fachhochschule Valais - health and social work.

Project "Prevention of the damaging effects of unemployment on the health of persons over 50 who are taking steps to be reintegrated": separate pilot projects with unemployed workers and advisors were started concurrently in the cantons of Geneva, Valais, Fribourg and Jura. The intention was to raise awareness of health and increase self-responsibility in health matters, as well as to find models of good practice and publish them (including training courses and information material).

4.4. Services

4.4.1. Swiss Re

In order to confront the increasing psycho-mental requirements and strains which are also affecting the private lives and/or the health of employees, early steps are taken to enable workers to find a healthy work-life balance in every stage of working life and prevent burnout. Risk management is preferred to case management.

4.4.2. Swisscom Fixnet

The project "50plus" is an answer to the human resource policy challenge of efficiently using the potential of older workers. Different career models are implemented and the necessary conditions for a gradual exit from working life are created through the use of age-related part-time work and flexible retirement models.

4.5. Regional projects

"50+santé"
Initiated by DiPPS Dispositiv Intercantonal pour la Prévention et la Promotion de la Santé (authorised cantonal agent for health promotion) this projects works for three years.

Involved are labour inspectorates, economic offices, social welfare offices, employer organisations, trade unions and companies; their work is inter-cantonal (Fribourg, Geneva, Jura, Neuchâtel, Valais and Vaud) and inter-sectoral together with the canton.

The aim is to enable persons of 50 and beyond to protect and improve their health potential.

The fields of action are conditions of life connected to work.

- Working conditions
- Unemployment
- Retirement.

Programme section - Create a heath promoting environment through:

- Health promoting activities for the over-50's.
- Work and health 50+ - from the fact to action.
- The key role of statutory measures.

Strengthen resources in connection with work:

- Reduce age related difficulties at work.
- Prepare for retirement and make the transition from work to retirement easier.
- Prevent or reduce the damaging effects of unemployment on health.

United Kingdom

John Griffiths

<table>
<tr><th>Field of promotion</th><th>Physical strain</th><th>Psyche / cognition</th><th>Mental / social competence</th><th>Professional competence</th></tr>
<tr><td>Action</td><td colspan="4"></td></tr>
<tr><td>Relief of physical strain / WHP actions</td><td colspan="2">Workplace health promotion measures *</td><td></td><td></td></tr>
<tr><td></td><td colspan="2">Behaviour-based measures *</td><td></td><td></td></tr>
<tr><td></td><td colspan="3">Assessment and management of workplace risks</td><td></td></tr>
<tr><td></td><td colspan="3">Developing sensible management practices on job design and workload</td><td></td></tr>
<tr><td></td><td colspan="3">Involvement of staff in workplace-based health improvement initiative</td><td></td></tr>
<tr><td>Age-related working hours</td><td colspan="3">Reducing working hours prior to retirement</td><td></td></tr>
<tr><td></td><td colspan="3">Abolition of fixed retirement age / implementing flexible retirement policy</td><td></td></tr>
<tr><td></td><td colspan="3">Developing sensible management practices on working hours</td><td></td></tr>
<tr><td>Qualification</td><td colspan="4">Equality of access to career change, advice, re-training and job-search support</td></tr>
<tr><td></td><td colspan="4">In-work training grant / support for continuous training / lifelong learning</td></tr>
<tr><td></td><td colspan="4">Stores with staff consisting only of 50+ers (e.g. B&Q)</td></tr>
<tr><td></td><td></td><td colspan="3">Exclusion of age criteria in recruitment schemes</td></tr>
<tr><td></td><td colspan="4">Allowing changes in levels of responsibility</td></tr>
<tr><td></td><td colspan="4">Workforce near retirement age coaches / mentors younger ones to impart knowledge</td></tr>
<tr><td></td><td></td><td colspan="3">Helping seniors to get self-employed</td></tr>
<tr><td>Communication</td><td colspan="4">“Age Toolkit” - diagnosis for profiling age within the organisation and identifying age related issues</td></tr>
</table>

Field of promotion	Physical strain	Psyche / cognition	Mental / social competence	Professional competence
	Inclusion of age diversity management			
	Promoting the benefits of employing a mixed-age workforce			
		Anti-discrimination policy on recruitment and retention (press, research, awards etc.)		
	Training on sickness absence management			

** Exercise, nutrition, consumption of alcohol and nicotine, relaxation*

Fig. 21: Summary of actions - United Kingdom

1. Political basis

1.1. The Code of Practice on Age Diversity

In June 1999, the UK government published a voluntary code of practice entitled "Age diversity in employment" together with implementation guidance and case studies to show how a number of employers have tackled age discrimination. The Code sets out the principles of good practice to be adopted in recruitment, selection, promotion, training and development, redundancy and retirement.

1.2. The government led consultation process on age diversity in the workplace

On July 2, 2003, the government published its consultation document, "Equality and Diversity: Age Matters" outlining proposals for outlawing age discrimination in employment and vocational training. The key areas covered are:

- direct and indirect age discrimination in employment and vocational training,
- recruitment, selection and promotion,
- different treatment on the grounds of age,
- mandatory retirement ages,
- unfair dismissal law, and
- redundancy payment rules.

The open consultation period ended on October 20, 2003, with the drafting of the legislation being undertaken during the latter part of the year and into 2004. A consultative process followed the drafting of the legislation and the legislation will be laid before Parliament in 2005, with an implementation date of October 2006. Prior to this the government will develop and publish guidance which will enable employers to prepare for the new legislation and individuals to familiarise themselves with their new rights.

2. National programmes / projects

2.1. New Deal 50 plus

New Deal 50 plus is a programme for people aged 50 or over that have been out of work and claiming benefits for at least six months. It provides:

- personal advice and support in finding a job,
- £ 1,500 in-work Training Grant,
- access to financial support when in work, paid as part of the Working Tax Credit. The amount depends on income and circumstances.

An employer who recruits an individual who is eligible for New Deal 50 plus may be able to access a government funded grant of up to £ 1,500 to help train the new employee. This can be used towards the costs of the individual gaining an NVQ (National Vocational Qualification), getting some computer lessons, going on a health and safety training course or any other work related training.

2.2. Age Positive

Age Positive is the government's campaign to promote the business benefits of an age diverse workforce to employers. Age Positive actually refers to a team working in the Department for Work and Pensions in Sheffield and London, responsible for strategy and policies to support people making decisions about working and retirement.

The Age Positive campaign promotes the benefits of employing a mixed-age workforce that includes older and younger people. They encourage employers to make decisions about recruitment, training and retention that do not discriminate against someone because of their age. They use publications, research, press, events and awards initiatives to get the message across - and to help employers prepare for legislation in 2006, to outlaw age discrimination in employment. They support a website full of every type of information that can help interested parties - be it individuals or organisations - access knowledge on age and older-worker matters.

The response from UK employers to the Age Positive initiative reveals that many of them are taking a very positive position on the issues surrounding the employment of older workers.

2.3. Third Age Employment Network

The Third Age Employment Network (TAEN) is committed to better opportunities for mature people to continue to learn, work and earn. The Network has a membership of 240 organisations and groups across the UK and provides cutting edge expertise in helping mature people overcome barriers of discrimination and realise their aims and ambitions. TAEN is a campaigning organisation, working with the media, employers and government to change attitudes and public policies. It does this by:

- representing the interests of all mature people who want to continue training and working, so that they have the opportunities to use their skills and experience in the economy,
- campaigning against all forms of age discrimination in employment and training, and achieving legislative recognition of age as a form of discrimination equal to race, gender or disability,
- creating equality of access for mature people to workforce development and services which meet their needs in career change, advice, re-training and job search support,
- aiming to be the leading centre of expertise and communication on age and employment, and
- supporting the Network of Members by sharing good practice, supporting new initiatives, signposting organisations and individuals, and campaigning on their behalf.

3. Players / national agencies

3.1. Professional organisations

3.1.1. The Confederation of British Industry (CBI)

The CBI's mission is to help create and sustain the conditions in which businesses in the United Kingdom can compete and prosper for the benefit of all.

They are a prominent lobbying organisation for UK business on national and international issues, working with the UK government, international legislators and policy-makers.

The CBI recognises that the drop in employment rates for the over 50's has serious negative consequences for individuals, employers, and society as a whole. It supports the Department for Education and Employment's Voluntary Code of Practice on Age Diversity as a means to challenge age stereotypes and encourage employers to review existing policies and practices.

3.1.2. The Chartered Institute of Personnel Development (CIPD)

The Chartered Institute of Personnel and Development (CIPD) is the professional body for those involved in the management and development of people.

The CIPD is committed to the removal of age discrimination in employment because it is wasteful of talent and harmful to both individuals and organisations. The use of age, age bands and age-related criteria reduces objectivity in employment decision-making and increases the likelihood of inappropriate decisions.

According to CIPD (among others), employment decisions based on age are never justifiable because:

- age is not a genuine employment criterion,
- age is a poor predictor of performance, and
- it is misleading to equate physical and mental ability with age.

CIPD believes there is an important business case for employers to take action to remove age discrimination and has undertaken research and published guidance to raise awareness. It is involved in educating personnel practitioners and employers about the issues. Although CIPD recognises that the law can help to effect change in employment practice, self-regulation based on increased understanding is favoured as the best way to encourage employers to deal with age discrimination.

3.1.3. Chartered Management Institute (CMI)

The CMI is a leading organisation for professional management representing 74,000 managers. The CMI strongly supports the view that age should not matter when making employment decisions and has taken an active interest in ageism for some time. In 1996 they undertook a major research project surveying managers' attitude to age and employment, and they have been actively involved in the DfEE's (Department for Education and Employment) working party for promoting diversity in employment.

The CMI highlight working conditions as an area that needs to be addressed in relation to older workers and state that many workplaces need redesigning by means of an ergonomic assessment. The CMI purport that action is needed to reduce the incidence of work-induced stress and musculo-skeletal strains as these are the most commonly cited reasons why older people leave work.

Current CMI research is focusing on the quality of working life and organisational health. This research will take a holistic view of workers quality of life. Age will be a factor which shall be cross-tabulated with other measures of quality of working life.

3.1.4. The Trades Union Congress (TUC)

Trade unions and the TUC are fully committed to the push to eliminate ageism at work. Trade unions are working constructively with employers to eliminate age bias in all employment policies and procedures. They have also welcomed the trend towards ending mandatory retirement, and have actively supported moves to do so in many sectors, particularly in the financial and retail sectors. The TUC is very concerned that the progress that has been made so far is maintained and built upon and that employers not see new age equality legislation as a threat.

3.2. Academic departments

Please note, the following list is not exhaustive, merely a selection of UK University Departments that are active in the field.

3.2.1. The Institute of Occupational and Environmental Medicine (IOEM), University of Birmingham

The mission of the Institute is to develop and conduct research and teaching programmes in occupational and environmental medicine, epidemiology, ergonomics, toxicology, hygiene, and other related disciplines in order to prevent health hazards in the workplace and in the common environment with an aim to create healthful general and working environments. The institute has a particular interest in the effects of age on work ability and associated occupational health requirements, and recently housed a seminar on "The Ageing Workforce".

3.2.2. The Institute of Work, Health and Organisations (I-WHO), University of Nottingham - the development of a national research agenda

The Institute of Work, Health and Organisations (I-WHO) is a postgraduate research institute of the University of Nottingham. It focuses on the contribution that applied psychology can make to occupational, environmental and public health and safety, and the management of related health services.

It is committed to the active promotion of "healthy work, healthy workers and healthy organisations". This mindset both drives the Institute's education and research agendas, and establishes the culture within which those activities take place. It has a particular interest in the interaction between work, ageing and health, and in particular, the issues surrounding the quality of life, health, and work performance of the older worker.

3.2.3. Centre for Research into the Older Workforce (CROW), University of Surrey

The Centre for Research into the Older Workforce was created in response to the growing policy interest in the ageing population and addresses the government's desire to encourage more people to stay in paid work later in life.

The centre is particularly interested in exploring the attitudes of older people and employers to retirement and work after 50, in how the skills of people over 50 can help overcome skills gaps and shortages, and in the kinds of education and training which might help. Their core research strategy comprises three broad research themes:

- Job design - How can work be reconfigured to make it attractive to older workers?
- Individual motivation - What persuades people to stay longer in work?
- Intermediaries - What kinds of training, advice and guidance are available to support people entering or staying in work later in life, and how effective are they?

3.3. Government departments

3.3.1. Department of Work and Pensions

Within the scope of its activities, the Department has a specific age related target to address, namely, "to increase the employment rate of people aged 50 and over, taking account of the economic cycle, and significantly reduce the difference between their employment rate and the overall rate".

This target fits into the government's overall strategy of tackling poverty and moving people into work. For older people this means resolving the various employment barriers faced by older people and includes:

- influencing employers by emphasising the benefits of a mixed age workforce through programmes such as the Age Positive campaign,
- the New Deal 50 plus programme for people aged 50 or over who have been out of work and claiming benefits for at least six months, and access to other employment programmes and initiatives,
- increasing the benefits of staying in work longer through increases to the rate at which people are compensated for deferring state pensions and by giving them the choice of a lump sum, and
- age discrimination legislation covering employment and training which will come into effect in 2006.

3.3.1.1. The Health and Safety Commission / Executive

The development of a long term occupational health strategy, "Securing Health Together" provides a framework for the issues of occupational health faced by all workers to be addressed, but also provides a unique opportunity to embrace the needs of older workers. Several groups were established with the goal of examining how the programmes could be achieved. One of these, the Support Programme Action Group describes a vision of a minimum level of integrated occupational health, safety, rehabilitation and job retention service established for all. The objective of such a service is to maximise the functional capacity of individuals, the organisations in which they work and the wider economy. The Group has also set out the need to utilise the ageing worker differently but effectively.

3.4. Devolved government

3.4.1. The Welsh Assembly Government

"The Strategy for Older People in Wales" was published by the Welsh Assembly Government in January 2003. The Strategy addresses an extensive range of issues with regard to older people including employment and health promotion and describes the ways in which the Assembly will act.

Employment figures very highly in the Strategy and is largely addressed in Chapter 5. One of the strategic aims of the chapter being to "promote and develop older people's capacity to continue to work and learn for as long as they want, and to make an active contribution once they retire". The strategic objectives which emanate from this aim include helping older people to set up their own businesses, with Prime Cymru (described in section 4.2.2.) being established as a result.

Health promotion for older people is also recognised as a key element in enabling them to remain active in all aspects of their community and in delaying the onset of, and reducing the impact of illness and disability.

3.4.2. The Scottish Executive

One of the main vehicles for addressing issues of health and employment in Scotland is the Scottish Executive's "Healthy Working Lives" Strategy, which has as its aim to "provide support and opportunities for individuals to maximise their functional capacity throughout their working lives".

It is recognised that employability is at the core of the approach, and consequently "Healthy Working Lives" addresses a wide range of issues associated with it such as:

- "Support for the development of basic skills for those who find themselves at some distance from the workplace,
- providing services to address physical or mental health conditions and advice on vocational, education or training issues,
- ensuring that people work in safe, supportive environments,
- enabling people to maintain awareness of the importance of healthy lifestyles, and
- providing people with access to a range of rehabilitation services should physical or mental health issues compromise effectiveness".

Age is encompassed within the Strategy which also acknowledges that the commitment of employers is essential, and that one of the ways of creating that commitment is to make and publicise the business case which will persuade employers to invest in creating and sustaining supportive and inclusive cultures. Other actions which are needed include:

- offering employment opportunities to disadvantaged groups,
- providing health benefits for staff, and
- promoting involvement in workplace-based health improvement initiatives.

The importance of occupational health services is highlighted in the Strategy where it notes, "it requires a comprehensive approach to the promotion and management of occupational health and safety within Scottish workplaces to retain and sustain a healthy, productive workforce".

Within the Strategy it is also noted that value of the workplace as a setting for the delivery of health promotion needs to be demonstrated and that this can be done by identifying the ways in which, "the workplace can be used to support national programmes on smoking, drugs, obesity, alcohol, physical activity, health and homelessness and mental health".

3.4.3. Northern Ireland Assembly (The Assembly was suspended on October 14, 2002, and talks are ongoing. The Secretary of State has assumed responsibility for the direction of the Northern Ireland Departments.)

The Office of the First Minister and Deputy First Minister have put out for consultation a strategy titled "Promoting the social inclusion of older people: Ageing in an Inclusive Society". This is the government's strategic approach to ensure that the discrimination older people may face in the provision of goods, facilities and services are addressed, and aims to help to support the legislative framework designed to protect older people's employment rights. The finalised report will be available in April 2005.

In Northern Ireland population trends indicate that there will be a substantial age shift towards older people over forthcoming years. These will inevitably have an impact on the labour market. Between 2001 and 2041, the number of people aged 50 and over in Northern Ireland will increase by 56 % from 485,000 to 759,000 people. During the same period, the older age group of over 70 years will more than double from 158,000 to 327,000 people.

One of the proposed five strategic objectives in the strategy will be to address comprehensively the economic and financial inclusion of older people. Under this objective the strategy proposes the following:

- ensuring that the pension system works as effectively and efficiently as possible for older people in social need,
- promoting of employment opportunities and entrepreneurship among older people,
- promoting of the role of older people in the Social Economy in order to develop business opportunities, employment and services relevant to older people, and
- developing opportunities for lifelong learning and skills in information and communication technology.

The full document can be viewed at www.ageinginni.gov.uk.

4. Projects

Many organisations in the UK are addressing the issue of the ageing workforce. The case studies set out below are drawn from the list of examples of good practice as identified by Age Positive (http://www.agepositive.gov.uk). In compiling this report each of the organisations below was contacted. No specific criteria for inclusion was used other than geographical location, i.e. the examples represent practice in England, Northern Ireland, Scotland and Wales.

4.1. Private sector

4.1.1. B & Q

B&Q is the largest home-improvement and garden centre retailer in the UK as well as in Europe, and the third largest in the world. The Company has had a long-standing positive approach to employing older people, having had a policy in place since 1990. Such a policy came about due to a need for alternative sources of labour following an aggressive expansion campaign, low unemployment in some areas, and high staff turnover, especially in the 18-20-year old sector.

A pilot study conducted in 1991, whereby one B&Q store was staffed entirely by over-50's saw 18 % higher profits, 39 % less absenteeism, and six times lower rates of turnover than other B&Q stores. Subsequently, B&Q have developed a range changes to the way it works including:

- the abolition of a fixed retirement age, and
- the exclusion of age criteria in any of its recruitment or training schemes.

The age profile of the workforce is regularly monitored and in 2003, 21 % of the workforce was over 50, with the oldest employee being 90 years old.

The Company takes an inclusive and individual approach with regard to employee health and well-being. Information is available for all employees about such issues on the company's intranet site. Managers are provided with training on sickness absence management and where and how to make reasonable adjustments to a person's work in order to respond to specific health needs.

4.1.2. The Royal Bank of Scotland Group

The Royal Bank of Scotland Group (RBSG) is one of Europe's leading financial services groups and the second largest bank in the UK.

The RBS group has sponsored an Age Toolkit - a diagnostic tool for profiling age within the organisation and identifying age related issues. It has used this toolkit to conduct a comprehensive age audit in order to assess market position, highlight existing issues, areas of good practice and areas for improvement. The results and analysis will help form the age diversity agenda and strategic planning.

The group is committed to retaining the talent and skills of its existing workforce and is currently developing a flexible retirement policy that will include options to reduce the number of hours worked and allow changes in levels of responsibility.

Analysis of staff retention issues by the group highlighted mature staff retention rates being higher, on average, than those of younger staff. This has resulted in an advertising campaign focused on attracting older applicants.

In addition, the group is currently developing its Health & Wellbeing strategy to ensure health services and benefits reflect the needs and challenges presented by an ageing workforce.

4.1.3. Westbury Homes

Westbury Homes is a house-building service. Older workers are employed in a wide range of roles at all levels in the company; a quarter of employees are over 50. Older workers are an integral part of the organisation, valued for the experience that they bring to the job and are able to impart to other colleagues, and their ability to relate to the house-buying client.

The organisation deals with employee health and well-being issues on an individual basis. All employees are subject to a risk assessment. Changes to work design such as ergonomic adjustments have been made in response to requests from employees. The company tends to respond to challenges as they arise, regardless of age.

Psychological well-being is inexplicitly maintained and promoted through a system whereby site managers who are approaching retirement are moved to coaching/mentoring roles to provide support and impart knowledge to younger managers. This assists in providing a sense of self-worth to older employees.

4.1.4. Ulster Bank Group

Ulster Bank Group is committed to ensuring that it can employ and retain the best person for the job and the importance of diversity in developing a workforce that reflects, and thus best serves, its increasingly diverse client base.

The Bank's Equal Opportunities policy ensures that employees are aware of its positive attitude to age diversity, and all recruiters are trained in equal opportunities. Currently there are 360 employees who are 50 plus, which equals 7.2 % of the total Ulster Bank population. The equal opportunities policy will help all employees to develop their full potential and will assure that age is not seen as an unnecessary barrier to recruitment, promotion or training. This will involve basing employment decisions on objective, job-related criteria, encouraging employees of all ages to develop their careers, ensuring that employees of all age groups participate in training and have the chance to improve their skills and experience, and avoiding assumptions about the physical abilities and career intentions of older job applicants or employees.

The Bank has a very comprehensive workplace health promotion programme in place and, while maintaining its statutory obligation, it seeks to promote health, safety and welfare as a continuous drive for best practice. There is a comprehensive programme of actively monitoring, measuring and reviewing all policies and procedures to ensure that they remain compliant with the relevant legislation.

In order to demonstrate its commitment to age diversity, work has already begun on formalising the flexible retirement policy, which will be communicated to employees in 2005. A "Wind Down to Retirement" policy has already been developed and is due to be implemented in the first half of 2005. This policy allows employees to reduce their working days/hours in a three-month period prior to retirement. It is envisaged that the new flexible retirement policy will explicitly link into the pending wind down to retirement policy.

4.2. Public sector

4.2.1. Bridgend County Borough Council

Bridgend County Borough Council is one of 22 local authorities in Wales. Serving a population of just over 128,000 it employs 7,500 staff and has been proactive in addressing the issues of an ageing workforce. The Council has a long track record in the development of workplace health promotion initiatives, twice being awarded the Welsh Assembly Government's "Health at Work: The Corporate Standard Award", given in recognition of an employer's commitment to promote the health and well being of its staff.

In terms of addressing the issue of age, a key step occurred in December 2003, with corporate endorsement of the Council's Age Policy. The policy provides a framework for equality and age diversification to be fully integrated across the Council.

Other steps taken by the Council include:

- complete elimination of the use of age limits and age ranges in job advertisements,
- development of an age profile of the workforce,
- inclusion of age diversity in the Council's Business Agenda,
- adoption of a flexible approach to retirement.

Through the work of the Training Teams, Manual Handling Coordinator and Occupational Health Services, older workers are provided with advice and guidance on workplace risks and ergonomic issues. Their work situation can be modified to address their specific health, safety, and well-being needs.

4.2.2. PRIME - Cymru

In Wales, an organisation exists specifically to promote the benefits of self-employment and provide professional support to people aged over 50 who want to start their own businesses. It encourages older workers to consider the opportunities that self-employment can bring and to channel previously gained work experiences into a new and challenging field.

PRIME-Cymru was formed in May 2001, following an enquiry from HRH Prince Charles, the Prince of Wales. The Prince's Trust helps young people form their own companies and the Prince thought an organisation providing similar practical support and encouragement for older people would be beneficial. PRIME-Cymru has so far helped establish over 800 new businesses. As a contributor to the Support Programme for Under-Represented Groups, it is funded in Wales by the EU (Objective One) and the National Assembly for Wales.

A similar organisation exists in England.

Summary

Christian Boukal, Oskar Meggeneder

Initial situation

Much is at stake in the years to come: economic prosperity, secure employment, a stable system of state care for the aged, the corresponding solidarity between the generations and the social peace resulting from this.

These goals will be difficult to achieve unless the effects of demographic change on the labour market are recognised. An ever decreasing number of young people are confronted with an ever increasing number of people in retirement, and the effects on retirement insurance and pension funds are already being felt, as are the effects on the availability of well-trained and experienced workers. The problem will not be solved by merely increasing the retirement age without taking steps to care for the health of these employees.

It is also becoming apparent that the change of paradigm from viewing age as a model of deficits to viewing age as a model of compensation is taking place, a change which has long since taken place in the field of science. Ageing no longer means that mental and physical abilities are reduced, but only that there is a change in them. It is true that physical strength decreases, but this is compensated for by mental abilities, which can even increase with age, given the right support.

Awareness of the problem

The intensive participation of ENWHP members in the compiling of this report shows clearly that for some time many countries have had an eye on the problem of a decreasing birth rate and an increasing lifespan with the above aspects in mind.

WHP has made indisputable advances in recent years - not least through the activities of the ENWHP - but also because the topic has been taken up by company advisors and representatives of interest groups. These groups obviously realise that demographic change is a problem they share, because in many countries representatives of both employers and employees are working together to find solutions. Where these groups are not actively working together, they are at least participating in talks on the subject.

However, within the partner states of the ENWHP there are different levels of knowledge and therefore differences in the number of proposals for solutions intended to buffer the labour market and pension systems against the problems expected.

Additionally, countries which have only recently overcome the effects of state monopoly on the economy have a different set of priorities and problems when compared to countries which have long enjoyed a social partnership.

The 5th initiative of the ENWHP focuses on helping companies and their ageing workers to keep fit and survive this time of demographic change by showing them various successful measures and initiatives. The partners of the ENWHP and the countries participating were required to document the legal requirements, the proposals of relevant stakeholders and any measures for older workers which had been successfully implemented in WHP. The aim was to compile a compendium for all those interested or affected which would provide an overview of all the measures and proposals in tabular form with an index.

Basic principles

Before the WHP actors can work on the problems, a consensus has to be reached on what the situation in companies really is.

This is the reason that all the partners give priority to the analysis and communication of problems connected with the coming demographic change. Analysis shows that working conditions must be orientated towards the special abilities of older workers if companies do not want to lose them - and their knowledge and experience - prematurely.

Methods and structures of communication ensure that both parties in the working process - employers and employees - feel sure that their problems will be heard and that agreement can be reached concerning the improvement of working conditions presenting a health risk. Additionally, it is important to provide reliable scientific information on ageing. The scientific change of paradigm from a deficit model of ageing to a model of compensation needs to be communicated even more effectively, despite the progress already made in its acceptance.

Improvements in working conditions presenting a health risk will not mean that behaviour-oriented measures can be neglected - which is in keeping with the holistic approach of WHP. Consequently, personal lifestyle during leisure time will also have to be modified. The problems of older workers do not stay within the factory walls. Problems at work, whatever they may be, are often taken home and have an adverse effect on family life. Information campaigns will not be limited to company premises, but will be heard on the radio, seen on TV, on posters, in doctors' surgeries, public places and in the homes of the people concerned. Examples of such approaches can be found in this report.

Even though the identity of the main groups requiring intervention may be obvious, analysis and communication are still the basic activities necessary to deal successfully with the problem.

If problems cannot be dealt with where they arise, there will be the danger that a social problem could develop, which, in the extreme, can only be counteracted politically and consequently by legislation. But conflicts on this level have an ideological nature, and negotiations carried out to protect the interests of a group of clients tend to delay - if not prevent - the finding of a real solution. This is one reason why organisations with a political background or representatives of certain interest groups are trying hard to find a constructive solution. If this is found, tried out and proves to be practical, it will be difficult to refuse it a legal basis, should this seem desirable.

Areas for intervention

When information about the problem and possible solutions has been communicated, then work can begin on dealing with real weak points in work processes and working conditions which are a health risk.

Three large areas for intervention became apparent during the work on this collection. Interventions in these fields could contribute to the well-being and job satisfaction of the workforce and therefore to the prosperity of the company. Firstly, there is the identification of situations at work which put a strain on health; secondly, there is the creation of age related working hours, and finally, there is the safeguarding and further development of vocational qualifications for older workers.

Work situation

These measures aim to provide relief from physical strain for the workers concerned, and it goes without saying that such relief also brings a psychological improvement in the workers' situation at home and at work. Ergonomic measures which go beyond statutory health and safety requirements are also detailed in this report. Special emphasis is put on proposals for physical exercise during working hours to keep body and mind vigorous and resilient.

Working hours

Physical relief can also be provided by arranging special working hours for older workers - for example, changes in the rhythm of shifts, shorter night shifts or even no night shifts at all for older workers have proved to have particularly positive effects on health and wellbeing. Many employees are prepared to forego part of their pay in exchange for such arrangements, so that there is no basis for the argument that these measures are uneconomical.

Qualifications

Resulting from the electronic revolution, a third group of topics requiring our attention has appeared amid the rapidly changing organisation of working conditions and processes. The knowledge a worker has about the complex work processes is the real capital of a company. If this knowledge were not passed on, every team would have to 're-invent the wheel'. The knowledge of older workers must be kept available through further training if it to be of use to the company in the future. This means that it is counterproductive not to invest in the training of workers after a certain age - the improvement and upkeep of qualifications must be continued until the end of working life.

As practice has shown, job and personal satisfaction increases when workers have the feeling that they are well-qualified and therefore needed at work. If an older worker has the opportunity to pass on his knowledge and act as a mentor to a younger colleague - particularly when this is done instead of some particularly exhausting task - both sides benefit. This again results in more job satisfaction and consequently greater personal well-being.

The many practical examples and the status many of the partners give these topics show that there is potential for development even in advanced age. This is indicated by the multitude of examples in the report which propagate life-long learning, teams made up of several generations working together, and the high status young workers give to instruction from their older colleagues.

Investment that makes sense

The fact that retirement is just around the corner does not mean that measures to improve the working conditions and health of workers may be omitted. Anyone who thinks that investing in this area is a waste of resources is misjudging industrial truths.

Practical experience and the good reputation a company has earned through the way it deals with the workers, who have very often risked their health in the company's service, make a responsible company into an attractive and trustworthy employer for young people. This is how an enterprise gains the reputation of being an employer worth identifying with.

Authors

Austria

Christian Boukal, born 1958, scientist in the field of journalism and communication sciences, department of health promotion and preventive medicine, Upper Austrian Sickness Fund (Oberösterreichische Gebietskrankenkasse), Linz

Oskar Meggeneder, born 1945, sociologist, social economist and political scientist, CEO Upper Austrian Sickness Fund (Oberösterreichische Gebietskrankenkasse) in Linz, president of the Austrian Public Health Association (ÖGPH)

Belgium

Veerle Hemans, doctor in physical education, ergonomist, research coordinator of Prevent, institute for occupational safety and health, Brussels

Karla Van den Broek, business unit manager of Prevent, institute for occupational safety and health, Brussels

Czech Republic

Alena Steflova, born 1955, physician, occupational medicine and public health specialists, World Health Organisation - Regional Office for Europe, Liaison Officer in the Czech Republic.

Denmark

Kurt Æbelø, born 1959, anthropologist, Head of National Centre for Workplace Health Promotion

Ervin Jensen, born 1948, engineer with speciality on economy, expert in labour market relations and business development, owner and senior consultant in Silva Gruppen

Finland

Riitta-Maija Hämäläinen, M.Sc., MPH, researcher at the Finnish Institute of Occupational Health in Helsinki

France

Marion Gilles, born 1975, production and organisation scientist, member of ANACT (French national agency for the improvement of working conditions) Lyon, Project "Ageing Management all along Life"

Michel Vallée, born 1945, psychosociologist and organisation engineer, social mediator, in charge of the "psychosocial project" in ANACT (French National Agency for the Improvement of Working Conditions) Lyon

Germany

Reinhold Sochert, born 1955, social economist, project manager at the BKK (Federal Association of Company Health Insurance Funds) European Information Centre, responsible for the projects carried out by the European Network for Workplace Health Promotion

Hungary

Gábor Galgóczy, born 1941, M.D., Ph.D., director of the National Institute of Occupational Health

Iceland

Ása Guðbjörg Ásgeirsdóttir, born 1967, rehabilitation counselor (M.A.) and M.S. in business - management and strategy, head of Department of Training and Information at the Administration of Occupational Safety and Health in Iceland.

Ireland

Nadia Clarkin, born 1961, occupational psychologist, Senior research consultant with the Work Research Centre in Dublin

Richard Wynne, born 1957, occupational psychologist, Director of the Work Research Centre in Dublin

Italy

Lamberto Briziarelli, born 1935, medical doctor, professor of Hygiene and Public Health, director of the Experimental Center for Health Education, University of Perugia

Giuseppe Masanotti, born 1968, medical doctor, specialist in Hygiene and Public Health, Ph.D. in Health Education, University of Perugia

Sergio Perticaroli, born 1948, engineer, director of the Documentation, Information and Training Department of the National Institute of Occupational Safety and Prevention

Luxembourg

Paul Weber, director of the Labour and Mines Inspectorate, Luxembourg

The Netherlands

Lenneke Vaandrager, nutritionist, Ph.D. in health promotion, former coordinator of the department of Work and Health of NIGZ and since March 2005, associate professor Public Health and Society of the Wageningen University

Elsa van der Maas, born 1977, Labour and Organisation Psychologist, project employee at the NIGZ - Work and Health in Woerden

Norway

Odd Bjørnstad, born 1946, graduate engineer and occupational physiotherapist, senior advisor at the National Institute of Occupational Health in Oslo

Poland

Krzysztof Puchalski, born 1960, Ph.D., sociologist, senior lecturer at the National Centre for WHP at Nofer Institute of Occupational Medicine, Lodz

Patrycja Wojtaszczyk, born 1978, political scientists, employee of the National Centre for WHP at Nofer Institute of Occupational Medicine, Lodz

Romania

Theodor Haratau, born 1968, medical doctor, executive president of Romtens Foundation, Bucharest

Spain

Mariá Dolores Solé, occupational doctor, Head of the Occupational Medicine Department of the National Centre of Working Conditions of the National Institute for safety and Hygiene at work in Barcelona

Sweden

Bo Hagström, born 1946, political scientist, regional director of the National Institute for Working Life - South (NIWL-South) in Sweden

Ewa Menckel, reseacher emeritus in work science at the National Institute for Working Life in Stockholm and professor Ph.D. in public health science at the University of Halmstad in Southern Sweden.

Switzerland

Joseph A. Weiss, born 1958, physicist, scientific collaborator at the State Secretariat for Economic Affairs of Switzerland (seco), Zurich

United Kingdom

John Griffiths, born 1956, public health consultant, managing director work2health Ltd.

Index

The following list gives a review of WHP measures for older workforce that are either suggested or already implemented in the respective partner nations of the ENWHP.

Whereas implemented **measures** are set in **normal** characters, ***suggestions*** in ***italics***.

Underlined words or **phrases** reproduce the exact term within the text and allow for a better search.

They measures are indexed by country – starting with Austria ending with the United Kingdom.

The abbreviations found in brackets indicate the countries by its domain name for the www (AT = Austria, DE = Germany etc.).

The numbers indicate the page where the information can be found.

Please note that some of the actions taken or suggested may be repeatedly quoted under different headings due to their nature covering more than one decisive area of intervention.

1. Relief of physical strain / WHP actions

1.1 Occupational medicine / OHS / mental health promotion

1.2. Personnel policy / human resource policy

1.3. Teams of mixed ages

1.4. Working conditions / work environment

1.5. Vocational tasks

1.6. Checks / audits / screenings

1.7. Senior sections

2. Age-related woring hours

2.1. Time reduction / flexible work-time systems

2.2. Shift work

2.3. Part-time work / pensions

2.4. Work-life balance

2.5. Recreation and holidays

3. Qualification

3.1. Knowledege transfer

3.2. Vocational training / vocational experience

3.3. Career guidance

3.4. Trainer / management

3.5. Special training facilities

4. Communication / interaction

4.1. Interpersonal communication / contact / prejudice

4.2. Mangement / personnel policy

4.3. Information materials / media campaigns

4.4. Seminars on the cause of WHP and problems of ageing

4.5 Surveys / studies

4.6. Quick-check / guidelines / MOGP

4.7. Corporate social responsibility

4.8. Age diversity management

4.9. National and regional structures